MIND GAME

MIND GAME

An Inside Look at the Mental Health Playbook
of Elite Athletes

JULIE KLIEGMAN

ROWMAN & LITTLEFIELD
Lanham • Boulder • New York • London

Published by Rowman & Littlefield
An imprint of The Rowman & Littlefield Publishing Group, Inc.
4501 Forbes Boulevard, Suite 200, Lanham, Maryland 20706
www.rowman.com

86-90 Paul Street, London EC2A 4NE, United Kingdom

British Library Cataloguing in Publication Information Available

Library of Congress Cataloging-in-Publication Data

Names: Kliegman, Julie, 1991– author.
Title: Mind game: an inside look at the mental health playbook of elite athletes / Julie Kliegman.
Description: Lanham, Maryland: Rowman & Littlefield, 2024. | Includes bibliographical
  references and index. | Summary: "In Mind Game, Julie Kliegman offers insight into how
  elite athletes navigate mental performance and mental illness—and what nonathletes can learn
  from them. She explores the recent mental health movement in sports, the history and practice
  of sport psychology, the stereotypes and stigmas that lead athletes to keep their troubles to
  themselves, the ways in which injury and retirement can throw wrenches in their mental states,
  and much more."—Provided by publisher.
Identifiers: LCCN 2023023910 (print) | LCCN 2023023911 (ebook) | ISBN 9781538168066
  (cloth) | ISBN 9781538168073 (epub)
Subjects: LCSH: Athletes—Psychology. | Athletes—Mental health. |Sports—Psychological
  aspects.
Classification: LCC GV706.4 .K57 2024 (print) | LCC GV706.4 (ebook) | DDC 613.7/11—
  dc23/eng/20230828
LC record available at https://lccn.loc.gov/2023023910
LC ebook record available at https://lccn.loc.gov/2023023911

To the psychiatrist who told me I'd be dead by now. I'm not.

Contents

Foreword ix

Introduction: Learning from Our Idols xv

Part I: Eyes on the Prize: How Mental Performance Shapes Athletes. 1

CHAPTER 1: Mentally Tough: The Stereotypes That Athletes Fight. . 3

CHAPTER 2: Looking Back: A History of Sport Psychology 21

CHAPTER 3: Science and Practice: What Mental Performance Coaches Actually Do. 39

Part II: The Megaphone: Speaking Out about Mental Illness . . . 59

CHAPTER 4: The Firsts: Trailblazers Who Came Forward 61

CHAPTER 5: Open the Floodgates: More Athletes Join the Cause . . 79

CHAPTER 6: The Greats Chime In: Anxiety and Depression amid a Pandemic. 97

CHAPTER 7: On Campus: The Push for Better Care at Colleges . . 117

Part III: The Diagnosis: Coping with What You've Got 137

CHAPTER 8: Substance Use: From Alcohol and Cannabis to Psychedelics 139

CHAPTER 9: Body Image: Eating Disorders in Professional Athletes 159

CHAPTER 10: Life Out of the Game: Injury, Absence, and Retirement. 177

CONTENTS

Conclusion: So What's Next? 193

Acknowledgments 205

Notes 207

Select Bibliography 221

Index 233

About the Author 247

FOREWORD

In photographs, you most often find me with a thousand-watt smile on my face. The truest expression of my joy. Mouth wide open. Damn near every tooth showing. Gums and all. Cheeks puffy. Eyes squinting a bit. I have to remember to keep them open while smiling so big.

Brave. Courageous. Authentic. Words often used to describe me.

As a social advocate for all things justice, I'm propped up as an example to follow. Be brave enough to come out as trans in a heinous sports landscape. Speak on issues and topics people don't dare bring up. Be at the forefront of social change, as many Black women have been before me.

As a professional athlete, I'm praised for overcoming adversity. Perseverance is held up as the ultimate trophy in my profession. Sports love a comeback story. One filled with heroic triumphs against all odds. The more you've overcome, the more beloved the story.

This book is not that sports story. It is a book about the messiness of being human. Often, we are sold this notion that athletes are somehow exempt from the struggles of being just another regular-ass person. Yes, we do pretty extraordinary things that the average person absolutely cannot do. We can run faster than most, jump higher, and change directions with precision. Our coordination is something to marvel at. Because of our ability to stand apart within sports, we are robbed of the simplicity and the empathy that life is hard and our mental health struggles are real.

We just happen to do our jobs in a public space under the bright lights of spectators.

People often want the comeback story, but they don't want the messiness it takes to get there. This is a story about mental health or, as Julie will elaborate on in this book, mental illness. What happens behind the scenes in the life of an athlete? How do we show up and perform at the scale we do? How can we be better supported? What happens when an athlete is struggling with mental health? Are the people around them adequately equipped to support?

I want to walk you through a tough stretch I was having and show you how people can support. This is what showing up has looked like for me recently.

The 2023 WNBA training camp almost broke me. As athletes, we've done things that are mentally, physically, and emotionally grueling, and they take something from us. A piece of us. The most jaded parts of me believe that professional sports and mental well-being do not go hand in hand because the demands are too high. You could argue inhumane, even. The most hopeful parts of me believe that we just need to keep allowing people to show up fully and support them along the way.

I have a skin condition called tinea versicolor, a common fungal infection in sports due to the heavy amounts we sweat. Suffice it to say that I'm often itchy around my elbow creases, shoulder blades, and outer thighs. On this particular day, I couldn't shake the itchiness. This particular week, actually. I kept waiting for my skin to calm down, thinking, *Wow, the temperature change really set me off bad this time around.* I started to notice an itchiness in places that don't typically bother me. My head, shins, stomach, neck, pretty much everywhere. I felt like I was breaking out in hives.

On our next road trip, I brought it up to my trainer. Insisting this is weird and not normal. She prompted me with some baseline questions about detergents and any dietary changes and then mentioned it might be emotional.

I paused and scoffed. Could I be so stressed out that my skin is yelling at me? I took some Benadryl and quickly found a reprieve for the evening.

A few days later, I was having one of the hardest mental health days in sports I've ever had. We were 10 days into training camp with about one and a half off days. If you don't know what training camp is like, let me explain. It's essentially boot camp. The intensity is extremely high. We practiced for about three hours—not including lifting, film, or pre-/posttreatment from the trainer. I would leave my house around 7:20 a.m. and arrive at the gym a little before 8. Change and head to the training room to warm my legs up and get some tissue work done. Around 8:30, after finishing up my ankle exercises, I'd head to the weight room to lift with our strength coach. Around 8:45 to 9:20, I'm doing squats, box jumps, dynamic explosive movements, getting stronger and quicker. Around 9:30, I head to the court to get pre-practice shots in with assistant coaches. Then at 10, we all gather to watch film before practice. From 10 to 10:30, we watch and discuss schemes from the day before. Get to see what worked well and what we need to improve on. At 10:40, we head out to the court to officially warm up for practice. This warm-up lasts about 20 minutes. Active stretching, muscle activations, jogging, and dynamic explosive movements get us prepared for the intensity of practice. At about 11, we finish and have one final player huddle where we encourage each other to have a good day. Boom, practice officially starts. We practice from 11 a.m. to 1:30 p.m. Practice is full of drills, shooting, full-court running, playing against practice guys, scrimmaging. At about 1:30, we finish, and small groups gather to shoot a bit more with assistant coaches. By 2, it's time to stretch, cool down, go to the ice bath, and begin the long process of recovery for your body.

You can imagine, after many days of this schedule, how the effects start to wear on you. Not to mention, I am trying out to make the team. On my particularly rough day, I was stuck in a spiral.

I parked my car at the gym, and as soon as I got out, I was flooded with intrusive, repetitive thoughts.

I can't do this. I can't do it. I can't. It hurts. I'm so tired. I don't want to be here. I'm so tired of feeling this way. Why do I feel this way? I don't want this. I just want to feel good again. Will this ever end? What time is it? Ugh, I have to go lift today, too.

Dread.

First, the drowning feeling, then the berating yourself for feeling that way comes next.

But Lay, you wanted this so bad. Now you're finally getting it and you're ungrateful. This is just how hard sports are! Did you forget or something? Maybe you just don't want it bad enough.

I slogged my way into the locker room, changed, and went to lay down on the treatment table in the training room. As soon as I looked my trainer in the eyes, the tears started to flow. She hugged me instantly, and I explained that I'm just so drained. Emotionally and mentally. I need a break. She said she understood and that I needed to give myself grace. I'm doing amazing. At that moment, I realized the deadline for the final roster was merely days away. I'm so anxious and triggered by being cut the year before that it's starting to really affect my ability to show up and be present.

I was having a tremendous training camp. My whole mantra coming into this opportunity was to be radically present, and up until that point, I had been playing with such joy and freedom. Truly soaking up every moment. But what happens when the moment is full of dread, hopelessness, and spiraling?

And then I remembered the intense itching I felt that morning. It was tied to my emotional and mental state. Fuck. I am indeed so stressed that my skin is screaming.

I left the training room. Time to go to the weight room. The show must go on.

I debated calling an old mental health professional on the three-minute walk to the weight room. Instead, I called my wife. No answer. She's in a meeting. Welp, just keep breathing, Lay.

I can't breathe, I can't breathe, I can't breathe. This will never end.

Layshia, you won't feel this way forever. It's okay. Hang in there, you can do this.

No, it's not okay. It just hurts too bad. I can't.

My legs keep moving as my internal dialogue is in a full-blown fistfight.

I got into the weight room and was instantly grateful there weren't a lot of people there. Just one teammate, the strength coach, and her intern.

She asked me how I'm doing.

"My mental health is shit today," I said. Tears welled up in my eyes. I was desperate to feel some reprieve. Carrying it alone is what kills us. She gave me a hug instantly, and my teammate came over and asked what's wrong.

I told them, "My mental health is *shit* today, and I'm sick of it. I want to feel better. I'm just so exhausted. I'm frustrated. I've worked so hard to get to this place, and I want to feel joy again. This is everything I've wanted, and I just feel terrible." They told me it's okay to cry. I let it out. Unfiltered. Grateful for the space to show up exactly how I am today.

People are very used to that thousand-watt smile and the energy I bring into whatever room I walk into. I show up genuinely. It's actually really difficult for me not to. On the days I'm really struggling, it can be damn near impossible for me to fake it.

The strength coach offered to modify my workout into whatever feels good to me. At that moment, she realized that my lifting weights in the state I'm in might not be the most beneficial. In fact, it would be detrimental to put my body under that level of stress. Instead, she offered me a yoga mat and an ear, and we did some simple mobility exercises as we talked.

I felt my shoulders drop a bit. I could breathe a little bit. I felt less alone than when I walked in that day.

As I walked back to the gym for practice, I was ashamed, and I regretted that now the coach will think of me differently for struggling. That I'm mentally weak. That it's a sign I'm not built for this. All terrible stories. Even though she showed nothing but kindness, empathy, and understanding. It is going to take a long time to undo the deep-rooted belief that struggling mentally means that something is wrong with you.

These are the stories that for so long have been used against athletes when we do open up and talk about our mental illness.

I believe this systemic stigma is one of our biggest challenges to overcome in the sports world. We need more coaches and people in positions of power to normalize that mental illness is a part of sports just as much as a rolled ankle, lactic acid in your legs, or a pulled muscle. If you play sports long enough or at a high level, you will experience an injury at some point. It is inevitable. A jammed finger, a stubbed toe, a torn anterior cruciate ligament, a concussion—something will happen. In the same way, we need it to be understood that you will struggle with mental illness at some point. You will have hard days. It's inevitable. Instead of being reactive, how are we proactively helping athletes prepare and endure the rigors of sports and being human?

My strength coach is a prime example of how we can support an athlete in the moment. First of all, she had built enough human rapport with me that I knew she was someone I could trust. When she asked me how I was doing, I knew I could be honest with her. When I did open up, she was able to hold space for me. As leaders in this industry, I ask, how are you showing up as a container for your athletes? Do you understand that part of your job is to support the mental well-being of athletes? I hope that you do and that, if you didn't know before, you take seriously the stories in this book to better understand that more of us than you know are struggling. We need support.

My athletic trainer deeply understands that the health of an athlete is a holistic endeavor. Since the start of training camp, she has been setting up an entire health network for our team. From a sport psychologist to a nutritionist and any other specialists we need to see. She's normalizing mental illness as an aspect of sports.

In all of this experience, I have learned that even when I'm struggling, I can show up. I can show up for myself by being radically honest.

A few days later, I walked into the weight room, and the strength coach asked me how I felt. I said, "I don't feel terrible today." We laughed and celebrated that win!

Get people who will celebrate that you're not feeling terrible on any given day. My plea is for you to be someone to whom people can say how they're really doing.

Layshia Clarendon

INTRODUCTION

Learning from Our Idols

You know your favorite athletes' origin stories by heart. Dunking on a toy hoop. Skating before they could walk. Getting cut from the junior varsity squad. But do you know their mental health origin stories—the events that prompted them to speak up? Michael Phelps had the luxury of a magazine interview. Years later, Naomi Osaka had a skipped press conference. Simone Biles had the twisties—in other words, the gymnastics version of the yips, wherein her mind stopped being able to tell where her body was in space.

Another Olympian, Raven Saunders, who was considerably less well known, had just a couple of wristbands (we'll get to those in a second). The Hulk, as she has long been called, had left her track and field career at Ole Miss a year early, in 2018. The up-and-comer's sudden departure came not even two full years after she took fifth place in the women's shot put at the Rio Games as a 19-year-old. Saunders was honored with a parade in her hometown of Charleston, South Carolina. But after that post-competition high came, she'd learn, a pretty severe low. It's a fairly common experience among Olympic and other elite athletes.

At the time Saunders dropped out of school, she'd been ready to kill herself. But just before she almost went through with it one day in January 2018, she texted her former therapist, who told her to hang tight.

The therapist helped Saunders check into a hospital, where she stayed for about two months. Although not everyone loves—or likes or even tolerates—psychiatric hospitalization, for Saunders, it was "the greatest experience," she told me in 2022. "I was tired of lying to myself. I was tired of thinking everything was okay when I knew when I went home and I had to close that door that I was struggling."

So those wristbands? Hospital bracelets. They jump-started her willingness to go public with her experience of mental illness. Saunders, diagnosed with anxiety, depression, and posttraumatic stress disorder (PTSD), had snapped a picture of her wrist at the time of her hospitalization and tweeted it two years later after reading a story of a college athlete who *had* died by suicide. "On 1/26/18 I was omw to carrying out an attempt to end my life," tweeted Saunders, whose following on the platform had crossed 30,000 people by early 2023. "If not for sending a text to an old therapist I would not be here rn. Everyday I live is a gift bc that day could've been my last."[1] In a reply, she added, "To everyone especially all my student athletes out there if you ever need to talk or feel that no one understands the pressures you're under my dms are ALWAYS open. It gets hard but I promise you it'll get better."[2]

* * *

Saunders did get better, but her story around mental illness, like most of ours—athletic superstars or not—hasn't been linear or smooth. Her second Olympic go-around, in Tokyo in 2021, came amid the COVID-19 pandemic. That time, Saunders earned the silver medal, outthrowing everyone save China's Lijiao Gong. The Hulk, by then 25, demonstrated atop the podium, forming an X with her arms above her head. She later described the symbol as "the intersection of where all people who are oppressed meet."[3] Saunders has gone on to advocate for not only mental health awareness, but also racial and LGBTQIA+ justice.

The medal marked a high moment for Saunders, but she almost immediately faced another tragedy: Her mother, Clarissa, died just two days after watching Saunders place second. She had been in Orlando at a watch party for her daughter, along with Raven's younger sister, Tanzania.

Raven described Clarissa's death as putting her at her "deepest level of hurt"—but this time around when things got tough, the athlete felt more equipped to move through and cope with her devastation.

"This is how life goes. Something's gonna happen, but whatever it is, I'll handle it," Saunders said, outlining her mindset leading up to the Tokyo Games. "And then [my mother's death] happened. And I was like, *Oh, we're going there.*" Saunders laughed to me in disbelief at the timing of it all. This go-around she was able to implement the techniques she'd been building up to take care of her mental health—what she wasn't equipped to do the first time around, when she was contemplating suicide three and a half years before. She checked in with her therapist immediately on returning Stateside, communicated with her family, and stayed aware of her triggers.

Saunders's story is not one of a fairy-tale recovery, a one-way trip from depression to perpetual happiness; rather, like most of what's collected in this book, it's about the difficult slog of surviving on a daily basis. By hearing from elite athletes like her, we can better understand their origin stories—and our own. Although I'm not an elite athlete myself (if only!), I can relate to certain aspects of these icons' journeys.

* * *

It's hard for me to remember life without mental illness. Growing up, I struggled with depression and would, about a decade after I first showed symptoms, be formally diagnosed with bipolar II disorder. That life-changing label, which I identified myself before any professionals believed me, came only after many bad—I mean truly god-awful—therapists. It came after stints on medication from pill-pushing psychiatrists that only exacerbated my symptoms and even a brief, terrifying stay at a psychiatric hospital in 2018, complete with at least half a dozen emotionally abusive mental health practitioners. One psychiatrist, after I left the hospital, even told me not to worry about how the psychiatric medications would affect my thyroid disease because none of that would matter once I killed myself. He saw it as inevitable. I hadn't even been suicidal when I checked myself into the hospital. (The details don't matter to people like him.) Years later, after a lot of hard work on myself, I feel much more clearheaded and steady, thanks also in large part to myself, a supportive close circle, a few drugs I had a hand in choosing, and my sweet gray-and-white tabby, Penelope.

If it's hard for me to remember a life without mental illness, it's downright impossible to remember a life without sports. Growing up, I became a superfan of the U.S. women's national soccer team, tennis stars like the Williams sisters, and the New York Mets (I know). I played travel soccer throughout elementary and middle school, as a left midfielder, before switching to cross-country and track in junior high. Sports were a refuge for me, as they are for so many. But they're also pressure cookers brimming with anxiety, self-doubt, and sacrifice. In sports, you're signing yourself up for private criticism and a whole lot of public scrutiny, even on the youth level (looking at you, parents and coaches). Surviving in that atmosphere was no small feat for me, a mediocre high schooler thrilled to have lettered as a freshman. (A particularly scrawny kid, I drowned in my varsity jacket for four years straight and also refused to button it up in the winter because it looked less cool that way.) That's to say nothing of what survival entails for those talented enough to compete and even excel at the collegiate and elite levels.

Then there's the matter of stepping away from sport. I faced down this fear earlier than most: My troubles with the posterior tibial tendon on the inside of my right ankle started when I was 14 and quickly worsened. Two surgeries and the resulting nerve pain, due to a nasty complication from the second surgery, effectively shut down my running career by age 16. There was no real inciting incident—no stumble I could point to, no nothing.

My transition from runner to spectator was not smooth. The constant nerve pain in my foot, which persisted until I finished college and finally found the right physical therapist, chipped away at my mental health, worsening my depression. Moreover, my main avenue for stress relief had disappeared. Not overnight but close. I'm told by experts that athletes who lose their sports can experience something akin to grief, as if they'd experienced the loss of a loved one. That's what it felt like for me.

Given my own experience, fierce competitors who persevere through challenges and contort themselves not only physically, but also emotionally and mentally, to be ready on game day have always grabbed my attention. Athletes are some of our most exalted role models and for good reason, many would argue—their feats are impressive as hell. But let's do our best to take them off their pedestals: We all benefit when we see athletes as fully formed humans, not superheroes. (Sorry, Hulk.)

* * *

In March 2020, one of those supposed superheroes grew worried. In light of the Tokyo Olympics' yearlong delay due to the COVID-19 pandemic, Michael Phelps was most concerned not about the logistics of athletes qualifying or their fitness or their delayed pursuit of gold but about their survival.

"I really, really hope we don't see an increase in athlete suicide rates because of this," the most decorated Olympian of all time said shortly after the novel coronavirus hit the United States in full force. It shut down not only the Games as planned, but also sports and many aspects of public life entirely. "Because the mental health component is by far the biggest thing here. This postponement is uncharted waters. We've never seen this before. It was the right decision, but it breaks my heart for the athletes." Were he faced with this challenge in his swimming days, "I would have unraveled," he added.[4]

Phelps knew from personal experience that mental illness is always a serious risk for athletes, pandemic or not. After just about every one of his five Summer Games, Phelps retreated deep into depression, he has said. He has even, as he shares often now, contemplated suicide. "I was always hungry, hungry, and I wanted more," Phelps has said. "I wanted to push myself really to see what my max was."[5] He was seemingly a god in the pool who was painfully mortal out of it, facing down his suicidal thoughts in private. He came forward about the full extent of his experience with depression and attention-deficit/hyperactivity disorder (ADHD) only in 2018, two years after his retirement from swimming. (He had begun slowly opening up before the 2016 Rio Olympics.)

Clearly, Phelps has survived and thrived, but not everyone fares as well. Among college athletes, for example, suicide is the third-leading cause of death, according to the NCAA. There's no evidence to suggest that elite athletes experience mental illness at a rate higher than the general population (a whopping one in four adults per year), according to the International Olympic Committee, but they stare down these problems with higher stakes and more public scrutiny.

In recent years, well-meaning fans, coaches, activists, and even athletes have showered a lot of praise on those who, like Phelps, are, as the media reports always say, "starting a conversation" around "mental health" in sports. Simone Biles. Naomi Osaka. Kevin Love. DeMar DeRozan. They and many others are doing excellent work in speaking up about their experiences when it matters most, on the world's biggest stages, but not a single one of them *started* a conversation; rather, they represent some of the latest, most high-profile entry points into an increasingly active dialogue.

In reality, the conversation we're having began, at least in fits and starts, decades ago. "The role of sport psychology is being embraced, and the role of mental health in athletics is being embraced more than I've ever seen it," said Chris Carr, the Green Bay Packers' director of performance psychology and the team's behavioral health clinician. "I just think the issue of mental health is not new." The term "mental health" has its place, and we'll use it often in this book, but it's all too often deployed as a euphemism for mental *illness*—a way of evading the severity of someone's problems and the associated stigma and systemic issues. It can also be a way of evading the fact that they're having problems at all. Sportswriter Louisa Thomas of *The New Yorker* has rightly called the phrase "so broad as to become, at times, unhelpful."[6] Kate Fagan, the Meadowlark Media (Dan Le Batard and John Skipper's venture) and former ESPN personality, once a college basketball player herself, agreed, telling me, "Even just saying mental *health*, it takes away the grit of everything we're talking about."

In fact, some who have experienced mental illness firsthand reject that terminology, along with the concept that they have any disorders, and use a different term altogether: madness. The Mad Pride movement is a reclamation project born in the 1990s in which people who have been treated and often wronged by experiences in systemic psychological and psychiatric care take back power for themselves and speak out about what they've experienced, often liberally deploying what many would view as taboo pejoratives, like "crazy" and "insane," to describe themselves. Some but not all in this movement reject the treatment of madness with drugs. Many have been force-fed them in the past after all. It's a good reminder to always center people with lived experiences in their own stories and talk about their brains using their own terminology. That's what I'll strive to do in this book.

For clarity's and sensitivity's sake, I'll stick with the more widely used mental illness throughout but always with madness in mind. And when I write about mental illness, I'm using the term fairly broadly. Most people first think of anxiety and depression, but conditions like obsessive-compulsive disorder (OCD), PTSD, schizophrenia, borderline personality disorder, substance use, eating disorders, and so many more are just as important to discuss. I'm also writing about not only what has been diagnosed down to the letter of the *Diagnostic and Statistical Manual of Mental Disorders* (5th ed.) (*DSM-5*), the bible for U.S. clinicians treating patients, but also anything athletes feel they have dealt with, whether or not an upstanding professional has deigned to put a tidy bow on it.

To truly focus on mental illness, we also need to broaden our scope far beyond cisgender, straight, white, wealthy athletes who often have the most privilege (and therefore, typically, the most robust safety nets) to go public with their struggles. This is not merely an exercise in praising Phelps and others for what they have done, although we'll certainly do that when warranted. It's about chronicling the movement and, in doing so, finding the hidden figures and illuminating their challenges. For example, there's pressure on queer athletes, especially in men's leagues, to stay silent about their gender identity and/or sexual orientation, and that can compound any existing mental health issues they experience. The NFL's Carl Nassib, the league's first out gay player, has said just that: "The first couple of days, being out and being the only out player, my body felt like Jell-O. I was very anxious. But now I wanted to get this over with," he told reporters in August 2021 about the news conference he was then sitting through. "I wanted to move on and I just wanted to have a lot of clarity. I feel better today. I feel better than I did yesterday and the day before that."[7]

Also, rookies getting settled in their first pro leagues, younger athletes, or Olympians who depend on sponsorships for their income may not feel comfortable coming forward about mental illness. Their finances and reputations are at stake. "We're at a point where now the greats, the Simone Biles, Derrick Rose, can come out and say that [they're struggling], but we're not to a point where Susie, who's competing in a bantam basketball under-six team, can come out and say, 'Oh, I need a break because of my mental health,'" said Krista Van Slingerland, who served as the mental health manager for Game Plan, Team Canada's holistic wellness program for Olympic athletes. "You have to work to that privilege, I guess, which is not really the way it should be."

Part of the reason that disclosures like Biles's and Osaka's make major waves are because they come from athletes of color—who face even more stereotypes and barriers to opening up than their white peers. "We're in a space where as Black people, either you are invisible and you are silenced in a space, or you are rendered superhuman, which also gives this notion of invincibility, that we don't have pain, we don't have emotion," Akilah Carter-Francique, then the executive director of San José State University's Institute for the Study of Sport, Society and Social Change, once said. "It's a devaluation of their humanity."[8] That can't-win dichotomy makes it tough sometimes for Black athletes and other athletes of color to share their experiences and advocate for themselves and others.

What we need now, as we grapple with how to support athletes dealing with a host of mental illnesses, isn't to start a *new* conversation—whatever that would be at this point—but to continue to carve new grooves in the existing one. In doing so, we can take action on what we learn from others to make sports more understanding and supportive for athletes struggling. How can we make mental health care, including therapy appointments and psychiatric medicines, more affordable for the most vulnerable athletes? How can we ensure that they have qualified professionals to speak to both inside the gym, employed by their team, and outside, wholly unconnected from their sport? How can we staff sports leagues with supportive coaches who won't emotionally, physically, or sexually abuse players, thus further jeopardizing their mental health? These are some of the current, pressing questions propelling forward our long-held conversation. Increased awareness of this conversation is wonderful, but it alone isn't enough. It's something that frustrates WNBA veteran Layshia Clarendon. "There's still so much shame and taboo, and there's more conversation, especially in the sports world, about 'mental health,' but it's like, dot dot dot," they said. "So, cool, it's a buzzword, let's say it. But I think this is where I struggled, is how do we actually change things to address mental health and help people be healthier?"

* * *

It's not that we, historically, haven't cared about athletes' minds at all as they dazzle us with their physical prowess. It's just that when we have, it's often been with an eye toward mental *performance*, or the practice of optimizing athletes' on-field product using techniques to shut down negative thoughts and build up mental skills. How can we squeeze every last drop of productivity and strength out of an athlete? If my quarterback meditates, will he focus better in the pocket? If my starting point guard practices mindfulness, will her peripheral vision on the court get sharper? These questions are indeed valid—famously, even LeBron James meditates—and they have a rich history rooted in science. We'll explore that in greater depth to better understand the mental side of the game and how it can help athletes to victory while teaching them to process their emotions in healthier ways. However, those questions surrounding mental performance shouldn't be our *only* areas of focus as we consider what goes on between athletes' ears.

Many mental performance coaches, including those who practice with professional sports teams, are not licensed psychologists or psychiatrists and are therefore not qualified to treat athletes for even common mental illnesses like anxiety and depression, though they're trained to spot the signs and refer struggling athletes to licensed clinicians. This is not to say that mental performance coaches don't have their place. They do, and a good many are quoted in this book. Just don't trust anyone who refers to themselves as a "sport psychologist" without having a clinical psychology background.

I aim to show that an athlete's work on mental performance is not synonymous with work to upkeep their mental health, though the two are intertwined. Solid mental performance techniques like mindfulness and meditation can take an athlete only so far if they don't also, in tandem, receive proper care for any underlying mental illness or the seeds of one. To understand, destigmatize, and offer support for what athletes go through, we must consider both concepts in concert.

Mental illness can make even the bravest, strongest athletes look decidedly vulnerable, an image that many of them—and in many cases, their coaches, front offices, and fans—would like to avoid at all costs. But it's important that we don't demand an unrealistic level of mental toughness from our athletes, even those at the highest levels of sport, like Phelps. Instead, we'll need to accept athletes for who they are and really hear what they're saying about their own struggles inside and outside of the game. Wading into the nuances will give us more complete pictures of athletes' minds. It'll give us more empathy for them—and, along the way, increase our empathy for ourselves in our hardest moments. Most important, it'll give us the tools to continue and deepen a lifelong conversation about what goes on in our brains and help us find strengths in the depths of our perceived weaknesses.

PART I

EYES ON THE PRIZE

How Mental Performance Shapes Athletes

Mentally Tough

The Stereotypes That Athletes Fight

THE IDEALIZED IMAGE ATHLETES LABOR UNDER AT EVERY LEVEL OF sport is not subtle: They must be big (but not too big!) and strong (but if female, not too strong!). They are tough. They are immune. They play through injury. They don't cry. The list goes on and on, but perhaps the most harmful of these ideals is this: Athletes never admit weakness. And they never, ever ask for help.

Tyler Hilinski, at one time about to be the starting quarterback of the Washington State football team, might've not gotten the support he needed for those reasons. His parents certainly believe that. He used to occasionally drop off a friend, whose mother had died, at a psychologist's office. But his parents said he never saw one himself. "Tyler's mind didn't think like that," said his father, Mark. "He would go, 'Of course [his friend] had to see somebody. His mother died. What's wrong with me? I've got nothing. I've got everything I've ever asked for.'" Not only did he apparently never see a therapist, but he also never told Mark or his mother, Kym, that he was struggling with anything. He never really seemed to tell anyone else, either.

Tyler, Mark and Kym's middle child, a sensitive kid by all accounts, died by suicide on January 16, 2018, following his redshirt sophomore season at Washington State. He had just spent a week in Cabo with his parents and brothers. They took all their meals together and hung out constantly. "Room service and sun," Mark said. "That was it." And then, about a week later, "he was gone," Kym added.

Tyler was later found by the Mayo Clinic to have had stage 1 chronic traumatic encephalopathy (CTE). Diagnosed only posthumously and found in a high percentage of college and professional football players examined, it's thought to be caused by repeated brain trauma, like concussions and other hits to the head. It's also linked to symptoms like suicidal ideation. He took a head-to-head hit about 100 days before he died and kept playing through it.

Even so, Tyler's parents still aren't sure why exactly he died. They choose not to blame football, a sport that runs in the family. (His older brother, Kelly, and younger brother, Ryan, both played college football as well.) But even so, Kym said, "I do think there's some connection there." NCAA chief medical officer Dr. Brian Hainline has warned, "Concussion may be the elephant in the room, but mental health is the single most important health and safety issue facing our student-athletes."[1] He took over in 2013 and immediately made mental health arguably the college sports governing body's top priority. It's hard, if not impossible, to separate mental health from CTE.

The same year Tyler died, Mark and Kym started Hilinski's Hope Foundation to honor him by promoting mental wellness in college sports. "Unless you're just crying in a corner all the time—and there is absolutely care needed for those student-athletes, obviously—we're trying to help the group that doesn't know . . . how to ask for help," Mark said. From talking to athletes around the country, the Hilinskis now more fully understand what Tyler was up against as a football player, not just physically, but also mentally. "All the student-athletes that we've met with," Kym said, "they always say, 'I am strong. I have to grind every day. I have to go to practice. I can't appear weak, 'cause that's not what we are. That's not what our fans want us to be.'"

Athletes like Tyler are not often the type to seek help. And when they do push past the harmful stereotypes they've internalized—suck it up, don't cry—to get mental health care, they're not, historically speaking, the type to be public about what they're going through. Mental toughness is theoretically associated with a ton of benefits for athletes—perseverance, optimism, strength, and courage, to name a few. But at what cost?

Mental toughness is a term I've written about for *Sports Illustrated*. It might sound meaningless when deployed by pundits looking for reasons to criticize "weak" athletes, but it's a scientific concept that comes with very real benefits for those who practice it on a regular basis. "It is a resource that could give you the skills to fight any adversity as you're moving from Point A to Point B," Andreas Stamatis told me in 2022.[2] He's an associate professor of exercise and nutrition science at the State University of New York at Plattsburgh who studies mental toughness and works with other researchers to come to a more universal understanding of the term. Stamatis pointed out that displaying mental toughness is positively correlated with better mental health, more self-compassion, and more success on the field.

* * *

It's no wonder we expect athletes like Tyler Hilinski to be mentally tough. College football in the United States, with ties to soccer and rugby, started up just four years after the end of the Civil War, on November 6, 1869, with a New Brunswick, New Jersey, clash in front of a crowd of 100 between Rutgers and the university now known as Princeton.

The style of play itself immediately and unquestionably resembled warfare, with big, strong men lined up in formation using brute strength to capture territory. Fittingly, too, for the war metaphor, a large part of the colleges' competitive spirit had centered on the stealing of a Revolutionary War cannon back and forth between campuses (until Princetonians cemented it into the ground). The bitter rivals were facing off in this new-fangled sport because, the story goes, Rutgers had lost to Princeton 40–2 in baseball, and the Scarlet Knights wanted to exact revenge.

Of course, there were major differences between that 1869 game and the modern-day competition. At that time, the game's main focus was kicks—not touchdowns (throwing and carrying were both illegal). But the aggression, to be sure, was there. In other words, absent a literal war, the sport became a suitable outlet for boys and men to prove their masculinity and engage in sanctioned violence. In fact, even the site of the Civil War's largest Union training camp—and Confederate prison camp—was eventually turned into a college football stadium for the University of Wisconsin, Madison.

A modern-day player, Gabe Marks, a receiver for Washington State from 2012 to 2016 who knew Tyler Hilinski, saw the parallels with no prompting from me. "Football is a very controlled version of warfare," he said. "And the players are soldiers in their own battalions, whether that's the wide receivers or the quarterbacks or the linemen. Doing a particular job to win a war, which is in a 60-minute time frame or whatever it is, you have a lot of the same experiences that you can only know if you've gone through it."

Even more than 100 years ago, the war parallels were evident and intentional. "Two rigid, rampart-like lines of human flesh have been created, one of defense, the other of offense," wrote University of California president Benjamin Ide Wheeler in 1906, "and behind the latter is established a catapult to fire through a porthole opened in the offensive rampart a missile composed of four or five human bodies globulated about a carried football with a maximum of initial velocity against the presumably weakest point in the opposing rampart."[3]

Like in war, there was death, too, in football, on both the college and the NFL levels, especially as the twentieth century wore on. The causes ranged from suicide to traumatic brain injury to spinal cord injury to cardiac arrest and more. Some of the deaths were a direct result of abusive coaching, tied to that same mental toughness stereotype. In June 2018, Maryland offensive lineman Jordan McNair, just 19, died two weeks after a spring workout. He had been hospitalized with exertional heat stroke. McNair had had trouble standing upright after a series of long sprints in the heat, and coaches didn't recognize the issue. The university accepted legal and moral responsibility for McNair's death and fired head coach D. J. Durkin. (Strength coach Rick Court resigned after being placed on administrative leave.)

It shouldn't take death to learn that there's a limit to the toughness of even the strongest athletes, that we can't ride them indefinitely without consequence. (And I'm not even sure we've fully learned that lesson. After all, Durkin, as of early 2023, was a defensive coordinator at Texas A&M. Court, meanwhile, landed a job as a director of strength and conditioning for a Michigan school district.) "We have historically devoted all of our time to improving the competitive 'hardware' of young athletes," wrote Jim Bauman, a sport psychologist who has worked at several Division I universities as well as with the United States Olympic and Paralympic Committee, "to the exclusion of developing their healthy 'software.'"[4]

Not all sports have such gruesome origin stories, but they, too, have a history of leaving coaches and fans with the expectation that athletes will cultivate and maintain polished exteriors. Tennis, for example, was invented around the same time as football (though its roots date back to eleventh-century France), with the first Wimbledon tournament held in 1877. There's certainly no tackling—and no contact whatsoever between players, save for a handshake at the net. And yet, in many aspects, the same expectations were foisted on them. Although women were allowed at Wimbledon starting in 1884, their image had to be perfect. They wore floor-length dresses, corsets, and hats. Men wore blazers and flannel trousers. Both looks give off the impression that even as they grunted and sweat, athletes were presentable and fit to be idolized. In football and tennis and across all sports, the notion, developed more than a century ago, persists that athletes must be put together at all times, whether going into a pseudo-war or suiting up in all white before the Queen.

* * *

As of a 2015 *Sports Health* analysis of an NCAA database, the suicide rate of college athletes (0.93 per 100,000 people) had been substantially lower than that of the general college student population (7.5 per 100,000) and other people of college age (11.6 per 100,000), but those numbers don't tell the full story of athlete vulnerability. Men in particular are at a high risk—especially football players and Black athletes, even though female collegiate athletes are thought to experience more symptoms of depression than their male counterparts. Overall, a quarter of college athletes are thought to experience depression (compared with 8.4 percent of U.S.

adults who have experienced a major depressive episode), according to the *British Journal of Sports Medicine*.

One major reason athletes are prone to mental illnesses like depression is that they tend to closely tie their identity to their athletic performance, good or bad. It's rooted in a concept called "identity foreclosure," discovered by clinical and developmental psychologist James Marcia and defined as the premature commitment to an identity without exploration of other potential roles they could play in life. "The individual about to become a Methodist, Republican farmer like his Methodist, Republican farmer father, with little or no thought in the matter, certainly cannot be said to have 'achieved' an identity, in spite of his commitment," Marcia wrote in 1967.[5] Many have built on the concept in a sport context, specifically measuring "the degree to which an individual identifies with the athlete role."[6] That means that when an athlete is cut from a team, gets injured, or retires, their identity is sometimes suddenly nowhere to be found, which leads to distress and a lack of sense of self.

At a young age, it can be somewhat advantageous for extraordinary athletes to foreclose on their identity—it helps them stay focused in competition, where they are typically far and away the best performer in their area, winning with great frequency. But as they age and become the world's top athletes, facing stiffer competition, they find that their entire identities are at stake every time they step on the court or on the mat. A loss could crush them.

Michael Gervais, a high-performance psychologist, said that a loss can actually induce a fight-or-flight response in an athlete. He's worked with the Seattle Seahawks as well as other athletes, like Olympic beach volleyball star Kerri Walsh Jennings. Gervais suggested that being an athlete is about juggling and maintaining different assets. "Like a diversified portfolio from a financial standpoint, you diversify your risk, and it's the same way that we want to help athletes to know that they are more than an athlete," he said.

Factors like gender and race often further complicate the notion of athlete identity. Take Carmelo Anthony, the 10-time NBA All-Star who grew up in Brooklyn's Red Hook housing projects and West Baltimore. When he played basketball in Baltimore as a boy with his older cousin

Luck, "Crying was not allowed," he wrote in his 2021 memoir, *Where Tomorrows Aren't Promised*. "As a matter of fact, crying was the worst thing you could do. We were men, and men don't cry."[7]

Chris Carr, the Green Bay Packers' psychologist, who himself was an offensive lineman at Division III Wabash College, said that stereotype is the reason he keeps up a group message thread with his football players and staff. About twice a month, he sends out articles featuring men, specifically, talking about mental health, along with relevant resources. "There's a lot of myths about male athletes in particular," he said. "You consider all the cultural issues that are occurring with our athletes, athletes of color. So we take all those things into consideration at the start of their therapeutic process."

For Anthony, his identity seemed to be wrapped up in not only his need to prove his masculinity, but also his race. As a young Black man, growing up in majority-Black neighborhoods, he faced all the stereotypes and pressures and cultural factors that come along with that upbringing. "If we look at the Black male, it's really tied into that notion of Black masculinity, of the physicality of it and the manhood that's tied into it," said Akilah Carter-Francique, who at the time we spoke was the executive director of the Institute for the Study of Sport, Society and Social Change and a professor of African American studies at San José State University. Carter-Francique was a college track athlete herself at the University of Houston. "Nothing can break you," she said. Non-white male athletes in football and basketball (no coincidence that these are commonly the revenue-earning sports) have been found to have the highest rates of identity foreclosure, having committed to sports without exploring other avenues. Along with that leap into a premolded identity comes the requisite toughness.

"Vulnerability was a big no-no in my community, and everybody was always okay with this," Anthony wrote. "I mean they might walk up to you saying things like 'I know what you are going through, I lost my brother,' or 'They killed my best friend,' 'My uncle died of drugs.' Even as they attempted to hug you, it was hard to get past that uncomfortable feeling of Why is this person being so nice to me, what do they really want? The type of trauma we had trained us to think that everybody around, for the most part, only wanted to take and never truly want to help. The trauma told us that those hugs weren't free. The shoulder people offered you to cry on wasn't free. Everything had a price. The only question was, were you willing to pay it or not?"[8]

Although athletic identity foreclosure is thought to be more prevalent in men than women, perhaps because professional careers in sports feel less attainable for women with far fewer spots available, female athletes experience the phenomenon in their own ways, with a unique set of pressures and stereotypes to conform to. Carter-Francique said that Black women in particular must confront stereotypes rooted in both racism and sexism. "It's the . . . caricature of the strong Black woman. Very strong, mentally tough, physically tough, doesn't let anything break her." Superstar athletes like Simone Biles and Naomi Osaka are defying the odds by speaking out about their mental health challenges just as their male peers like NFL quarterback Dak Prescott and NBA guard and forward DeMar DeRozan are, too.

But athletic identity foreclosure is not limited to just Black athletes. Kate Fagan, who wrote the book *What Made Maddy Run*, about the 2014 suicide of Penn cross-country and track runner Madison Holleran, experienced it during and after playing basketball at Colorado Boulder in the early 2000s. She detailed that in her memoir *The Reappearing Act*. Fagan, who is white, occasionally experienced anxiety and panic attacks connected to basketball. "It was the age-old issue of my identity was tied to my performance, and those things are so intertwined to the point where really the numbers on the box score dictated my mental and emotional well-being," said Fagan, the Meadowlark Media personality. "And no one back then—and this was 2002, 2003—was using the language we're using now about identity and outside validation. No one suggested to me that I should focus on validating my self-worth with things that were in my control."

* * *

There's a very real expectation of perfectionism throughout elite sports. U.S. Olympic gymnast McKayla Maroney knows this idea perhaps better than anyone. She's faced a lot of scrutiny online for years simply for having a face. Her "not impressed" expression went viral after she received a silver medal on vault at the 2012 London Olympics. (That iconic face, which was immediately memed into oblivion, is now on a non-fungible token she released, because of course it is.)

The truth is that while Maroney was honored to medal individually and grateful to be in London with her teammates, with whom she won gold, she really wasn't impressed with *herself*. In fact, she was struggling. Maroney had fallen on her second vault, the finals of which are extremely flawed, as they don't allow for much warm-up time. "It's really unsafe," Maroney said. She did only about 40 vaults the entire time she was in London, what she called "the minimal amount" of practice. Plus, she was coming off a month of competing on a broken foot, suffered on a beam dismount while she had stress fractures because a coach urged her to push through jet lag and pain after arriving in London. (She wasn't even set to compete on beam at the Olympics.)

Athletes like Maroney face not only the internal pressure to be perfect, but also the objectification and expectations of fans who expect perfection themselves. Hainline, the NCAA's chief medical officer, said, "We objectify them and worship them. We can objectify them in the worst of ways. We see them as being different, as being mentally tough, as being able to get through all odds. . . . It's this idea that athletes aren't allowed to be vulnerable."

When Maroney, then 16, made That Face, which lasted only a couple of seconds, the public couldn't have known that she was having a deeply rough time underneath. "I was miserable most of the Olympics because of how much pain I was in," she said. On top of that, she said that Larry Nassar, the since-convicted team doctor, had been sexually assaulting her at the Games—the extension of a crime that had taken a toll on her mental health for years already. Her team may have won gold together, but "I just wanted a moment to myself that was triumphant in a way at the Olympics, and I didn't get it," Maroney said. "And yeah, I felt not impressed. I felt kind of dead inside about the whole experience there."

Then Maroney had to deal with the social media fallout. Fans expected perfection of her in not only her routines, but also her emotions. In their eyes, she had failed them. "At the time I was looked at as a bad sport, as spoiled, a bitch," she said. Now some have been more understanding since hearing her full story of that time period in her life and the public reckoning with Nassar, who is in prison for life for assaulting her and hundreds of other gymnasts. But the damage, in many ways, was done. She went from a few thousand Twitter followers to about 400,000 due to the meme, she estimated, a great many of whom bullied her relentlessly. She got death threats. She met then-president Barack Obama and had the strength to poke fun at herself, making the not-impressed face with him. People then misconstrued Maroney's tweet about it, which she posted before the photo came out, and thought she was *actually* unimpressed by the commander in chief. So she got more death threats.

Maroney has dealt with depression and anxiety since she was a teenager—specifically, since Nassar started abusing her. "Depression suppresses joy," she said. "If you're suppressing your anger, if you're suppressing all these things, it also turns down the volume on your happiness, on your joy. You can't just turn down one emotion. You're turning them all down." It's impossible for Maroney to decouple the abuse from her mental illness, and the negative social media attention from "fans" who expected perfection exacerbated everything.

Taylor Ricci can relate to the pressures of perfectionism as an athlete, especially as a gymnast herself. She competed at Oregon State and said, "You go into the competition floor, and your job is to seduce the judge and try to get that perfect 10.0." Her anxiety and depression only ramped up following a teammate's suicide. "I was not really able to process anything, whether it was joy or anger or sadness," she said. "And that feeling of nothing was more painful than any other feeling I've had."

Along with Oregon State soccer player Nathan Braaten, who had also lost a teammate to suicide, in 2017 Ricci founded the campus group Dam Worth It, dedicated to raising awareness of and ending the stigma of mental illness in sports. It was just two months before Tyler Hilinski died less than 500 miles away. "I was a full-ride scholarship student-athlete. I was doing well in school. I had all this support athletically, academically," Ricci said. "I was doing the sport I loved while getting an education, competing in front of a bunch of fans. And in my brain, I was like, okay,

I have all of this. Who am I to struggle with mental health when I have all these resources and supports around me? I think that's a big thing for a lot of athletes. We expect ourselves to be perfect like we are on the competition floor or on the game field, but we are scared to show that more vulnerable or weak side."

Ricci was so scared, in fact, that when she started going to see a mental health counselor on campus outside of the athletic department, she would hide from view her backpack with the word "gymnastics" printed on it, sometimes leaving it in her car just to ensure that none of her peers would learn that she, an athlete, needed help, too. After a couple of months of therapy, though, she began wearing her backpack into the counseling office with pride.

Another collegiate athlete, Mackenzie Morse, grew up without mental health on her radar at all. She didn't even think of her heroes as full people—just athletes. U.S. women's national soccer team superstars like Mia Hamm and, later, Abby Wambach were "these star-studded idols." She said, "I didn't know who they were as a person, but all I knew is I wanted to be like them. *Oh, Abby Wambach has short hair? I'm going to have short hair.*" It's the equivalent of a first grader thinking that their teachers sleep at school.

Morse, a Dartmouth ice hockey and rugby alumna now in her late twenties, works for the U.S. Olympic and Paralympic Committee as a manager of athlete outreach and engagement. She has also consulted with her alma mater's women's lacrosse team on managing their mental health, and she runs "The Sideline Perspective"—a blog where athletes share their experiences about being "sidelined" from their sports—whether due to injury, the COVID-19 pandemic, or retirement. But it took her years and years to see that mental health was worth focusing on in both her idols and herself: "Even through college, I don't think I really thought of athletes having mental health struggles because I spent the first two to three years of school denying my own, and denying my own because I thought they weren't right to have," she said. The main issue she struggled with was disordered eating characterized by a fixation on healthy eating. It all goes back to wanting to be the perfect athlete.

***

The pressure to be perfect—and perfectly tough—comes not only from fans and the players themselves but from their coaches as well, whether or not they realize it. They control so much of an athlete's career, from whether they get significant playing time to how hard they must work in practice to whether they might get waived from the team or traded. "For them to say, 'You know, you just have to tough it out or suck it up,'" Hainline said, "I think that's a very hard stereotype to get by."

The WNBA's Layshia Clarendon (who uses all pronouns) said that who their coach is plays a big role in their mental health during any given season. She's had good coaches and bad, and she can feel the difference emotionally. Clarendon also references the National Women's Soccer League, where nearly 10 years in, in 2021, players had begun a reckoning, speaking up about abusive coaches on several teams and getting many of them fired. "It's not only the sexual abuse. It's the emotional abuse. It's the power dynamic," Clarendon said. "I think there needs to continue to be work around and transparency around who we're hiring, why people are let go, how they're operating within their jobs."

What constitutes emotional abuse in sports is not as clear as what constitutes emotional abuse in an ordinary workplace, Clarendon pointed out. "Sports is so blurry in that way. We're getting screamed at and we're in close quarters with each other in really intimate settings that are different than being in an office space," he said. "Physical boundaries are a lot closer. All those things within sport make it a very difficult work environment where you have to be very intentional, and you need people with a lot of integrity to operate within these spaces."

Clarendon hopes that the future of mental health care for athletes will include leagues and front offices taking a hard look at who is allowed to coach and why. They also want to see a streamlined system for players to anonymously file complaints about those coaches who have crossed a line and damaged their players' mental well-being. The demographics in coaching, Clarendon said, should also continue to shift away from being mostly white men. In the WNBA, for example, there's always talk around the need to hire more female coaches and Black female coaches in particular—after all, the league itself is mainly Black and female. We're used to talking about the importance of diversity in coaching from a social justice and equity perspective but not from a mental health perspective, Clarendon argued.

When it comes to broaching mental health issues with coaches, players may be inclined to sidestep the issue entirely—and many coaches are happy to do the same. "The traditional idea has always been, 'Don't talk about it, because he's going to get worse,'" St. Louis Cardinals manager Oliver Marmol has said. "That's not the answer. The player knows he has a problem. The coach knows he has a problem. But then there's this rule. *Let's not talk about it so it doesn't get worse.* And it's like, dude, it's serious. But there's always this divider, where the coach knows, and the player knows, but nobody talks about it."[9] Perhaps it's more comfortable to sit in silence—but for whom? The player certainly doesn't benefit. The coach likely does: It's one fewer issue to deal with and one way they can perpetuate the illusion that strong people never need help.

It's hard to imagine that coaches, once they do know about a player's mental illness, can completely stop themselves from factoring it into their game-time decisions. "You're on a team of 20, 30, or 100 people, if you're a football player, and you're fighting for that spot on the field or on the competition floor," Ricci said. "You know there's that fear, that stigma where I say if I'm struggling with my mental health or I'm struggling with anxiety or depression, that Coach isn't going to play you." Mark Hilinski said he's seen the phenomenon, too. "We still know there are coaches that just simply don't believe," he said. "They don't think mental health is an issue. They think there's tough people and weak people."

Many coaches aren't ready to meet the moment society has reached in the mental illness dialogue, Fagan pointed out. "The euphemism of old-school coaches, who know they have to say the right thing but kind of roll their eyes at this quote-unquote next generation mentality still exists," she said. "And then I think anyone who is alive in the world has gotten whatever messaging they've gotten about what depression or mental illness might look like, and it could just be self-conscious. Well, then, are coaches doing their own mental health work and are they really checking their reaction if an athlete of theirs shares something about whatever it may be? Are they really on a day-to-day basis checking themselves that they're not treating that athlete differently?"

* * *

The professional mental health guidance that Josie Nicholson received as a soccer midfielder turned striker at Loyola University New Orleans was unhelpful, to say the least. She was struggling with alcohol use in the mid-1990s. Her counselor, not in the athletic department setting and not at all fluent in athlete culture, said something like, "I see that you try to be tough. You don't have to be tough in here." Nicholson's internal reaction was swift and sure: "Bitch, please." Followed by, "I'm not trying. I just am." The counselor proceeded to advise her to quit soccer, "the one thing that was keeping me getting out of bed in the morning," Nicholson said. After a late night at the bar, Nicholson's teammates would find her and make sure she reported to practice.

Nicholson's negative experience with college counseling explains why she has a more progressive way of working with today's athletes as an assistant athletic director for sport psychology at Ole Miss. She also runs a podcast, *UNIT3D*, with the Hilinskis. When students come to her saying they can't cry or they have to stay tough, she listens, first and foremost. Nicholson sits with them in the weight of that stereotype and learns from the student instead of dismissing their mindset out of hand. She wants to know how a certain stereotype has served an athlete throughout their life. For example, what does someone gain from not crying in public? There must be value in the wall the athlete is upholding. "It's not breaking [the stereotype] down," she said. "It's not getting behind the wall. It's saying that wall doesn't have to be mutually exclusive to vulnerability because both can exist at the same time."

Other retired athletes are similarly trying to coach the next generation to sit with complex emotions rather than seeing them as incompatible with toughness. Kelsey Neumann is deliberate about how she teaches her fourth graders about mental health. They won't all become athletes, she knows, but they can all learn the lessons she picked up as an ice hockey goalie in college and for the Premier Hockey Federation's

Buffalo Beauts. She has each of her students at St. Christopher Catholic in New York decorate a goalie mask to represent who they are. It's a fun art project that's also meant to convey the idea that everyone wears a mask of sorts and that, when lifted, you see that person's true feelings and emotions. She hangs the masks on her classroom's front door.

"All of us have feelings," Neumann often reminds her students. "All of us have emotions that we don't always understand, we don't always get." It's a message that Neumann, who experiences anxiety, depression, and ADHD, didn't have reinforced for her in the sports world growing up. She played hockey on boys' teams and lacked a female mentor on the ice. "It was always that 'toughen up, don't let them see you sweat' kind of mentality," she said. "Being the only girl, you definitely didn't want them to see you cry, because that could be a sign of weakness." As a coach today for youth goalies, who often bear the brunt of parents' anger and their own self-blame when their team loses, she wants to give kids, especially girls, a more emotionally open experience.

Kids today are also fortunate to grow up in a world where *The Weight of Gold* exists. The HBO documentary, released in 2020 during the heart of the coronavirus pandemic, was executive-produced and narrated by Michael Phelps. It's an eye-opening look at the mental health challenges Olympic athletes face, with their identities wrapped up in sports and their quests for medals. It features household names like hurdler and bobsledder Lolo Jones, speedskater Apolo Anton Ohno, and skier Bode Miller.

Jones, for example, outlines the suicidal thoughts she used to have, a symptom of her PTSD from tripping over a hurdle at the 2008 Beijing Games. She couldn't go to the grocery store without people bringing up her fall. She'd be driving and secretly hoping a truck would hit her and end it all. Jones, who I've spoken to for *Sports Illustrated*, was one of several athletes in the documentary who opened up about suicidal thoughts and the other costs—emotional, physical, and financial—of being an athlete. It's stories like those that crack the image that Olympians and other elite athletes are as perfect as they seem.

The documentary could've been transformative for young athletes like Morse had it existed when she was growing up. "Maybe instead of

10-year-old me thinking Mia Hamm couldn't possibly ever want to get married or do anything outside of soccer, maybe a 10-year-old swimmer looking up to Michael Phelps sees that and is like, *oh, okay, I get that Michael Phelps is a swimmer, or was, and is also all these other facets of a human*," she said. "[The film] gets to burst that bubble earlier on than mine was."

There's also fictional media like *Ted Lasso*. The Apple TV+ show, which debuted in 2020, chronicles the story of the titular character, played by Jason Sudeikis, as he leaves the comforts of U.S. college football behind and travels to England to tackle his first soccer coaching job, for AFC Richmond. Billed as a fish-out-of-water comedy with the obvious U.S./U.K. gags, it quickly became so much more. Centered on the emotions of Ted, his boss (Hannah Waddingham), and his players, it's a show about navigating and working to eliminate toxic masculinity from sports and from life. Wrapped up in that pursuit is the characters' mental well-being.

In season 2, Ted, who had begun experiencing panic attacks (see the stellar yet unfortunately named season 1, episode 7, "Make Rebecca Great Again") amid a tough first season abroad and a divorce he never wanted, grapples with seeing the team psychologist, Dr. Sharon Fieldstone (Sarah Niles). He is resistant at first, determined to keep up his cheery, resilient facade. Over the course of the season, though, as he continues to unravel, he puts his trust more fully in Dr. Sharon. It's revealed by season's end that Ted's father killed himself when Ted was a teenager.

The show reminds us that even our toughest, most upbeat athletic figures require a little help sometimes. "The fact that [Dr. Sharon's] a main character in one of now very few sports shows, I think is reflective of the moment in a new and refreshing way but is also just accurate in terms of what athletes and sports teams have been trying to implement for a long time," said Mike Delayo, a Penn State graduate student researching the rhetoric of popular culture through sport. As a high school baseball player, he himself would shake with anxiety while at bat. The earlier athletes understand the mental and emotional toll sport can take, the better they can set expectations for themselves and also discover other facets of their identities.

* * *

It's clearly harmful to stereotype athletes as being unusually mentally tough, which may prevent them from coming forward to disclose mental illness or whatever else they may be struggling with. It's also, Neumann argued, pretty harmful to do the exact opposite: idolize athletes who choose to share their struggles with us. She wants fans and the media to reach a point where it's not "an *Oh my god, did you hear that [NHL goalie] Robin Lehner came out and said he has bipolar? Or Oh my gosh, did you hear that so-and-so has ADHD or anxiety?*" That approach, she stressed, is oversimplistic. An athlete is just living their life and navigating a fairly common and ordinary illness that others face all the time. "It brings light to the subject, yes, but at times I feel like it's saying here's a way that this person is completely different from everyone else," Neumann said.

Athletes aren't automatically "brave" for pushing through mental illness to do their jobs and live their lives. "It's more like, *Oh, they have that too? That's cool,*" Neumann said. "I wonder if their story can relate to my story." That's one productive way to move the mental health conversation forward: hearing out an athlete, considering their story, assessing where we have common ground with it, what we can learn from, and where we can help. That area in between being exalted as superhuman for being tough and being exalted as superhuman for being vulnerable is going to take a massive cultural mindset shift to pinpoint. To understand where we're going, it helps to first understand the origins of sport psychology and the way we have historically thought about (or not thought about) athletes' mental health.

CHAPTER 2

Looking Back

A History of Sport Psychology

ONE OF THE OLDEST ROOTS OF SPORT PSYCHOLOGY IS IN A HUT IN THE
Alps. In 1894, an Italian physiologist named Angelo Mosso climbed
Monte Rosa with his brother Ugolino, a professor of pharmacology, an
army surgeon, a medical student, and 10 Italian mountain soldiers, whom
Angelo referred to as his "humble comrades."[1] After the ascent, which
took about 24 days, the group stayed in a hut at 14,960 feet for 10 days,
fewer than was desired due to lung inflammation of one of the soldiers.

As chronicled in the excellent prehistory and history of sport psychology called *Psychology Gets in the Game*, the participants were required
to lift dumbbells and have their physiological and biochemical measurements taken. The resulting study, published three years later, revealed that
the person leading the mountain climbing group fatigued more quickly
than his peers. There was also a rivaling effect between the soldiers: Especially when they were bored, they had the desire to compete with one
another in weightlifting tests.

Mosso's study doesn't exactly resemble what we think of as sport
psychology today. So many athletes—from the youth level all the way
up to LeBron James—now tout the benefits of the field without having
scaled a mountain to test their respiratory function at altitude. For example, there are mindfulness apps aplenty of varying quality and endorsed
by your favorite athletes. As Mosso and a handful of others show, sport

psychology is not at all a new-age phenomenon; in some form, it dates back to the 1890s, albeit with many stops and starts along the way.

"I think part of what sport psychology does is it just centers more of a more scientific attitude towards sports in general," said York University psychology professor and *Psychology Gets in the Game* coeditor Christopher D. Green of the importance of the profession. "It cuts through—whatever we call them now—old spouses' tales that scouts pass on from one to another, and they carry a certain kernel of truth but they're kind of missing the bigger picture." In other words, sport psychology supplies the method behind coaches' madness.

Norman Triplett, who is often (erroneously) credited as the founding father of sport psychology, published one of the first such studies in the field. It would take the better part of a century after that before the profession really took off. Triplett was a graduate student at Indiana University. A star sprinter as a kid, he grew up to play on the faculty basketball team of Kansas Normal School, an institution for training teachers, and advise the track team for 30 years. But much of Triplett's professional work had nothing do with sports. He merely dabbled in the field, without making a point of returning to it. Also, he did not have any students to take after his interest in sport psychology.

Here's what Triplett did do in the sports realm, though: In 1898, he published a study as part of his master's research at Indiana in which he measured times for cyclists who raced alone versus cyclists who competed against others. Those who had competition raced faster, he found, at an average of 5.15 seconds per mile, up to 25 miles. It seems like common sense now for anyone who's even attempted *Mario Kart* solo, but at the time, it wasn't widely known as the principle of social facilitation, a social psychology concept. The study was published in the relatively popular *American Journal of Psychology*.

Multiple sports-related studies came before Triplett's: Philippe Tissié's, Edward Wheeler Scripture's, and Mosso's. Tissié, a French physician, was also much more well known for his work outside of sports: He is credited with discovering the concept of the "mad traveler," or someone in a fugue state. And like Triplett, he took a particular interest in cycling—more specifically, in his case, the psychological phenomena of training and competition as well as the therapeutic use of sport and exercise to combat psychopathological disorders. In 1894, Tissié published "Observations physiologiques concernant un record vélocipédique," or "Physiological Observations Concerned with a Cycling Record," in which he noticed that factors like hope of success, self-reliance, and spectators' enthusiasm can all improve performance. He also showed that in long-distance races, emotional regression to primitive states was possible along with experiences like hallucinations.

Scripture, meanwhile, is also most famous for something outside the field of sport psychology. In an 1895 book, he coined the term "arm-chair psychologist."[2] But the year before, the U.S. physician and psychologist had published a study about fencers' reaction times and movement speeds. Novice and expert fencers had the same reaction times, but experts had quicker movements. Like Tissié's work, Scripture's wasn't published nearly as prominently as Triplett's, in this case relegated to his own journal, *Studies from the Yale Psychological Laboratory*, which he stopped publishing in 1902.

By 1900, on the heels of those studies, there was growing recognition that sport psychology mattered. A Frenchman named Pierre de Coubertin, the founder of the International Olympic Committee and its second president, deemed psychology important to the Olympic movement given the rapid spread of sports. "These days the physiological effects of sports are studied in great detail. Curious experiments are being conducted that will fully elucidate that matter," he wrote in "La psychologie du sport," according to a 2000 English translation. "But the psychological side has remained in the shadows."[3]

Thirteen years later, Coubertin started the first sport psychological conference, in Lausanne, Switzerland. The intent of the three-day event, in his words, was "to make known a new science, or more exactly a branch of science which is unknown up to now by the public: the psychology of sport."[4] A paper by none other than Teddy Roosevelt was read to about 400 delegates on May 8, 1913, about the psychological benefit of sport. (He was unable to attend.) In particular, the former president praised boxing as a formative experience for him while criticizing its brutality and betting.

That conference could have marked the beginning of the rise of sport psychology in Europe and even the United States—but alas, the surge was still decades away, mostly because the practitioners thus far had few students to sustain commitment to the field. The 1920s, however, did see some progress. At the start of the decade, two researchers—Robert Werner Schulte of Germany and Petr Antonovic Rudik of Russia—established the first sport psychology labs. For many casual sports fans in the United States, though, their informal introduction to the field would come via the Babe.

***

George Herman Ruth Jr. was not best known for his lab results connected to early sport psychology. The Bambino, of course, was a star for his home run prowess and the curse that his sale from the Red Sox initiated. His two-way pitching and hitting abilities have been exceeded in Major League Baseball (MLB) only recently by Shohei Ohtani. On September 11, 1921, a *New York Times* headline blared, "Ruth Supernormal, so He Hits Homers." The subhead stressed that his coordination of eye, brain, nerve, and muscle was "virtually perfect."[5] This was concluded after just about three hours Ruth spent in a lab with sportswriter Hugh S. Fullerton at Columbia University's Morningside Heights campus, not far from Polo Grounds, where Ruth's Yankees then played.

Fullerton, a founding member of the Baseball Writers Association of America, escorted Ruth there on a hot summer day with the hopes of figuring out why the megastar was so successful at the plate and whether there were "other Ruths" out there to be scouted.[6] Researchers Albert Johanson and Joseph Holmes obliged, running all sorts of tests with all sorts of zany-sounding equipment hooked up, including a Hipp chronoscope on his bat and a kymograph on his torso. One test involved Ruth's swinging a 54-ounce bat (much heavier than bats used today) connected to wires to measure his breathing. Another involved Ruth's tapping a metal plate with a stylus as quickly as possible for one minute.

Fullerton published his results in *Popular Science Monthly*. "His eye, his ear, his brain, his nerves all function more rapidly than do those of the average person," Fullerton breathlessly gushed of how Ruth compared with previous test takers. "Further, the coordination of eye, ear, brain, and muscle is much nearer perfection than that of the normal healthy man."[7] The researchers who conducted the test never published the results in any professional journal. In 2006, writing for *GQ*, Nate Penn observed that in hindsight, the *Popular Science* write-up read "as a slightly laughable mixture of hero worship, hype, and sham science." And yet, as a peak performance expert told Penn, "in terms of testing and conditioning, baseball today is in the Dark Ages. In fact, the Babe Ruth testing was more appropriate and more intensive than anything any professional team is doing right now."[8]

Biographers would barely mention Ruth's foray into sport psychology, and his sitting for a battery of tests did not apparently inspire similar tests on other superstars. The tests Johanson and Holmes ran on Ruth weren't replicated on another MLB player until 2006, when St. Louis Cardinals legend Albert Pujols, for Penn and *GQ*, sat in a lab at Washington University in St. Louis. The results, apparently, were comparable, though Pujols never necessarily bought into the whole psychology aspect of it. "Psych tests are nice, but Albert just cares about baseball," his agent at the time told Penn.[9] While Ruth was testing, another baseball legend—this one in the field of sport psychology itself—was gearing up to leave his own footprint on the sport—and all of sports.

* * *

Coleman Roberts Griffith was born on May 22, 1893, two years before the Babe, in Guthrie Center, Iowa. His family moved often, including stops in California, South Dakota, and Illinois. He attended Greenville College in the Land of Lincoln as an undergraduate from 1911 to 1915, joining the University of Illinois for graduate school a year later after a teaching stint at Greenville. An active man with, by all accounts, a wry sense of humor, Griffith took frequent fishing trips and vacations to the wilderness. Although his early studies focused on topics like rats' fear of cats and rats' sense of balance, his life's work would eventually come to be defined not by rodents but by sports.

By 1918, Griffith had started conducting psychological studies, which would remain unpublished, on human athletes. He, like many of his predecessors, studied reaction times, in this case in Illinois football players. Griffith found that practice squads with quicker reaction times were more successful on the field, grabbing the attention of coach Robert Zuppke and director of athletics George Huff.

Before too long, Griffith started a version of his Introduction to Psychology course specifically geared toward athletes. ("The purpose of this section was to teach the facts and principles of introductory psychology by drawing upon athletic competition rather than upon daily life for illustrative material," Griffith wrote in 1930.[10]) It would be followed in 1923 by a course called Psychology and Athletics, the basis for his 1926 book *Psychology of Coaching*. (Sample line from chapter 1: "Ferocity and viciousness were the attitudes of the old athlete; high spirited sportsmanship and mental staying power or morale are the virtues of the modern athlete."[11])

Around the same time as Griffith was forming his specialized courses for athletes, his work got the (brief) *New York Times* treatment, on page 30, in April 1922. That's how novel his work was on a national and even an international level, that merely employing the use of psychology in a sports context was worth a write-up, with no findings yet to speak of. The news was that he had been appointed to Zuppke's advisory staff and that his research was expected to have implications for which athletes were selected to compete in baseball, football, and track at the university.

Griffith's Athletics Research Laboratory at the University of Illinois, part of the institution's new athletic complex, was the first in North America. He had big dreams for the lab, which encompassed two rooms totaling 1,050 square feet of space—complete with a rat colony—nestled on the second floor of the men's gymnasium. The sports to be studied included basketball, soccer, gymnastics, baseball, football, track, golf, swimming, and diving. The list of potential research projects included studies on general health conditioning, sleep, the learning of habits, the effects of drugs and emotional stress on athletic performance, and sex differences. The lab was approved in September 1925 and would exist only until 1932, but even so, it marked a much longer lasting foray into the field than those of researchers who had come beforehand in the United States and abroad.

An associate professor by 1925, Griffith won a Guggenheim fellowship that year seemingly unrelated to sport psychology. He left town in 1926 to start his studies in Berlin before his lab had published any results. It's unclear what came of his fellowship and how much of the proposal he actually completed. "He wasn't just making it up out of thin air," said Green, who has studied Griffith at length. "He was probably working on all kinds of stuff, but not as much of it was completed as you would have thought from some of the stuff he wrote." Back in Illinois in 1927, Griffith began publishing the following year, but his work didn't often appear in academic journals. When it did, it consisted of literature reviews or short, technical pieces as opposed to original research. So most of his reports were targeted more to coaches, not psychologists. (It's unclear whether this was his intention or whether scholarly journals of the time were reluctant to publish on sports.)

"The thing he was trying to impart on coaches was that there's this really important psychological aspect to athletic performance," Green said. "It's not just running and lifting weights. It's not just physical. You can get people into top physical shape, but if [they're] not mentally prepared for the rigors of the game, they're not going to perform at their best. . . . The way you get them to perform at their best is teach them how to focus, how to handle stress and anxiety, how to handle the mental aspect of the game. And coaches weren't prepared to do that."

In 1932, Griffith's lab was shuttered. There are two theories as to why, one being that it was simply a casualty of early Great Depression cutbacks by the university and the other being that Griffith had lost the confidence of Zuppke. He took up a different position at the university as the director of the Bureau of Institutional Research, which reported its collected and analyzed statistics on matters like teacher-to-student ratios and teaching load directly to the university president. But the closure of the lab would not mark the end of Griffith's time in sports.

* * *

Ahead of the 1938 baseball season, chewing gum magnate and Chicago Cubs owner Philip K. Wrigley reached out to Griffith about joining the team part-time. So Griffith hired an assistant (John E. Sterrett, a collegiate football and basketball coach), purchased at Wrigley's expense more than $1,500 (the equivalent of more than $28,000 today) of equipment, packed up, and headed off to Santa Catalina Island, California, for spring training. It was likely the first time a psychologist had worked with a professional sports team for any significant amount of time.

Hiring Griffith to sort out which qualities could predict success in major league players was probably a better idea for Wrigley than some of his previous ones. There was the time earlier in the 1930s when he paid $5,000 to a person meant to represent an "evil eye" to lay curses on other teams' batters. Wrigley also offered $25,000 if the club won the pennant. Nevertheless, the Wrigley–Griffith partnership was far from an easy win for either party—in fact, it wasn't even really a win.

The films and measurements that Griffith and Sterrett took of players on Santa Catalina Island don't exist anymore; what's left is a series of reports the two wrote for Wrigley throughout the 1938 season and, to a lesser extent, 1939 and 1940. There's also correspondence between Sterrett and Griffith that sheds light on the challenges they were up against, especially in team manager and former player Charlie Grimm. "I am convinced that Grimm is knocking our work as much as he can," the assistant wrote his boss early in the 1938 regular season, after the California getaway, on April 26. "Everything we say or do is reported to him and these are, in turn, passed on to the players. Grimm said to one of the players that he was afraid we might say or do something worthwhile and that if the players or the head office knew about it, it would put him in a bad light."[12]

The public perception of Griffith and Sterrett's work was seemingly no more charitable than Grimm's. In sportswriter Peter Golenbock's 1996 book *Wrigleyville*, he clearly outlined the issue with the owner's business model writ large. "With Philip Wrigley cutting off all avenues of improvement, the team's destiny was assured. He wouldn't spend money, wouldn't build a farm system, wouldn't listen to his baseball people. The Cubs would continue to remain competitive only so long as the players inherited from William Wrigley and [club president] William Veeck stayed healthy and didn't age and retire or if they weren't traded away foolishly. Both circumstances occurred."[13]

Golenbock seemed to share the belief that half a century earlier, Griffith's hiring was ludicrous. "Also harmful were P. K. Wrigley's quirky ideas. What the Cubs desperately needed was an influx of new, young players, but rather than take the steps to ensure that, P. K. Wrigley determined that the key to winning was not the hiring of scouts to bring the team talent but the hiring of Coleman Griffith, the director of the Bureau of Institutional Research, to study the reflexes of his players in order to determine their skills."[14] The reaction from the team, as chronicled by Paul M. Angle in his 1975 biography *Philip K. Wrigley*, was brutal: "The older players treated them as if they were typhoid carriers."[15]

Griffith had few kind words in return for the franchise that employed him. In July 1938, he criticized the spring training sessions as being "aimless, disorganized, and unproductive." He calculated at one point that each player spent only 47.8 minutes per day on practice that was "effective for the playing of baseball."[16] That came after months of writing reports advising Wrigley and Grimm to focus more on training. He suggested changes that were not, by any stretch, radical, like modifications to the game of pepper (a warm-up in which a player hits soft line drives at teammates standing nearby), a reorganization of batting practice, and more bunting, among other things. Sterrett abruptly resigned in mid-August to take a job coaching basketball at St. Louis University.

Despite the dysfunction, there was *some* good news for the Cubs ahead: In mid-July, Grimm was ousted as manager in favor of catcher Gabby Hartnett. The team rode that renewed spirit all the way to a National League pennant that fall before getting swept by the Yankees in the World Series. Despite the tension between Griffith and the team (though Hartnett was possibly more cooperative than his predecessor), Wrigley offered him a full-time job for the following season. Griffith declined, not wanting to move his family to Chicago, but stayed on part-time for two years. The number of Griffith's reports dwindled. Of the two managers Griffith worked under, Green said, "Finding the idea of a scientist coming in to tell them how to play baseball, they found that pretty threatening and they were unwilling to go along with it."

It would seem that Griffith never quite reached his ultimate goal: to determine what makes a major leaguer successful and how to scout for it based on a man's skills and reflexes. If the way Wrigley and Veeck told it is to be believed (and it probably shouldn't be), at one point near the end of the 1938 season, Griffith selected a group of younger players he'd been working with all summer to face a team chosen by the scouts. The scouts' team apparently "clobbered" Griffith's, Angle wrote, and eight or 10 of their players eventually made it to the high minors, while none of Griffith's did.[17] It's worth noting, though, that Green couldn't confirm the game ever happened, and Griffith's son didn't remember it, either. In fact, the Cubs didn't have a minor league farm system at the time, though the game *maybe* could have taken place between independent minor leaguers in theory.

Either way, the failed psychology experiment was "not unlike Wrigley's studies of workers to see if chewing gum could make them more productive," Angle wrote, summing up the mess. "But Wrigley was dealing with ballplayers, not factory workers. The Cubs players saw Wrigley's scheme as harebrained, and they refused to cooperate. When the Chicago press found out about it, Wrigley became a laughingstock, and Coleman Griffith disappeared as fast as he had come."[18] Griffith might have disappeared, but others eventually followed, making their own lasting marks in professional sports.

* * *

Speaking of laughingstocks, a man apparently without a doctorate degree improbably would become one of the next faces of sport psychology. Green, likely restraining himself, called this man "kind of a flimflam artist." But as Alan Kornspan, a sport psychology scholar, pointed out, "[David F.] Tracy's texts, and the things that he wrote about [sport psychology], were very similar to what we talk about today."

In June 1949, Tracy was at a New York City restaurant next to a lecture hall with other psychologists soaking in the air conditioning when a reporter, Claire Cox of the United Press Association, asked him whether psychology could be applied to baseball players. Yes, he said. He had worked with actors, radio commentators, and musicians, so why not athletes? Cox then asked whether he could work with a whole team at once. He replied, "Yes, it's better that way."[19] He didn't put much thought into telling Cox names of two teams he'd most like to work with: the Philadelphia Phillies or the St. Louis Browns. The conversation ended quickly and was forgettable for Tracy.

To his surprise, three days after the talk with Cox, Tracy found newspaper clippings in his mailbox, including "Psychologist Offers Services to Browns" and "Doctor Thinks Browns Need Help." Then, in September, Charlie DeWitt, a co-owner of the Browns, gave him a ring. Once Tracy got past what he thought was a prank call, he set up an appointment to meet with DeWitt the next day. They spoke of two semipro pitchers Tracy had been hypnotizing—yes, hypnotizing—twice a week. (Tracy, who was a medical student before World War I, had begun hypnotizing people during the war at a U.S. Army hospital in London.) DeWitt was reluctant to bring Tracy on in the middle of the season, but reporters inevitably caught wind of the meeting, and one of them, Bob Cooke, sports editor of the New York *Herald-Tribune*, encouraged him to give Tracy a shot that next year. "The eyes of the entire sports world will be focussed on the Browns," Cooke apparently told DeWitt per Tracy's retelling in his fascinating 1951 memoir *The Psychologist at Bat*.[20]

A few months later, at the winter meetings in New York, DeWitt and his older brother and fellow Browns co-owner, Bill, brought their wives and team manager Zack Taylor to dinner with Tracy. Of the five, Tracy hypnotized four right then and there, one by one, at their request. Normal stuff. Only Bill DeWitt held out. But he called the next morning and on hearing that his wife, who had had a headache, and sister-in-law, who had had shoulder pain, slept well, was sold. "You certainly performed miracles with them, and I hope you'll do the same for the Browns," Bill told him. That was the thing about hypnosis, at least as Tracy applied it: It could be used to treat any number of ailments or improve performance in any number of ways. It doesn't even always seem as if Tracy and his subject set an intention for the session beforehand.

The skepticism from outsiders came fast, even before Tracy rode the train with the team from St. Louis to California in March 1950. "The newspaper reporters landed on me as if I were a $100,000 rookie," he wrote. "With only a few notable exceptions, the reporters called me everything from a fake and a phony to a 'hypnotist with a magnetic eye.'" Within the clubhouse itself, too, trouble arose immediately. After Tracy had arrived in St. Louis on February 20, the DeWitts and Taylor set clear boundaries: He could not attempt hypnosis on the field, he was not a coach, he was not to sit on the bench with the guys, and he could not even so much as talk to them during games. This, of course, frustrated Tracy endlessly. "My job, it was turning out, was to perform a few psychological miracles on the Brownie players, hypnotize them in front of newspaper men, get write-ups in the papers and perhaps sell some season tickets," he wrote. "Psychology was to effect a vast improvement—at the box office."[21]

Despite his misgivings about the job, Tracy did not waste any time hypnotizing the Browns. He first selected Owen Friend, a six-foot, 23-year-old second baseman who had been called up to the majors on the last day of the 1949 season. Tracy told him his hands had magnetic powers, and he used the power of suggestion: Friend stood with his back toward Tracy, who told the player that "as I drew my hands past his head he would feel an invisible force pulling him back into my arms." Then the second baseman apparently fell back "almost immediately."[22]

Tracy then had Friend face him and told the player he would be unable to unlock his hands without getting permission. Then Tracy did what we always imagine hypnosis to be. He told Friend that his limbs and the rest of his body were growing heavy and that he was falling deep asleep. "At that time," Tracy wrote, "his eyes closed shut and he went into a deep hypnotic trance." He told Friend that while in the trance, he would be unable to move when awakened until given permission. Friend, once awake and apparently immobile, told Tracy, "Doc, I want to learn this—this is terrific."[23]

After Friend, Tracy proceeded to hypnotize seven more guys on that first morning. As the Browns performed well in spring training, the DeWitts were satisfied with Tracy—or perhaps just satisfied with the publicity he generated—and asked him to stay on through at least the first month of the regular season. The hypnotizer, for what it's worth, seemed to acknowledge the limits of his craft: "No amount of psychology is going to make a .300 hitter out of a .220 hitter, or a slugger out of a chop hitter, or a slick fielder out of an average shortstop. All psychology can do is help a natural .300 hitter to develop his latent ability and actually hit .300."[24]

Throughout the season, Tracy bore a weight on his shoulders. He felt like the sole representative of "Psychology," with a capital "P," in baseball, and like the DeWitts and Taylor had nothing to judge him against since no one other than Griffith had worked with a professional club. He also felt like Taylor saw him as just "about a step above the bat boy."[25]

But other coaches did seek out and value his advice, Tracy wrote. In hindsight, he theorized that a couple dozen baseball players, many of whom came in very nervous, would be more successful with a "managing triumvirate"[26]: a bench manager, a field coach, and a psychologist, all on equal footing. He also thought that starting with minor leaguers would prove a more effective strategy.

Tracy moved on after the 1950 season, taking up a short-lived job with the NHL's New York Rangers that November. On game day, he put the whole team under hypnosis before the matchup and in between periods. The slumping team lost that first night Tracy joined, 4–3 to the Bruins, but the Rangers felt a sense of improvement. Captain Frankie Eddolls apparently told a reporter, "That Doc Tracy was just what we needed. Our fellows were tense and pressing too hard. I really think he was able to help us relax."[27] The Rangers did not, however, keep Tracy on board.

As with Coleman R. Griffith, it's hard to say what effect Tracy truly had on the team—and he knew it to be true, writing, "If anyone were to ask me: 'Was your experiment with the Browns a success or a failure?' I frankly wouldn't know exactly how to answer."[28] But his effect on the field of sport psychology was more noticeable. His work was thought to inspire other coaches to take an interest in the field and connect with other, more legitimate and experienced psychologists. For example, Bruce Ogilvie, a pioneer born in 1920 who would become a key player in sport psychology in the decades to come, reported that coaches began approaching him after Tracy's highly publicized work. (Ogilvie went on to advise multiple professional sports teams. He was also an Olympics consultant for almost half a century.) Other hypnotists would follow soon after in baseball and other sports, including swimming, boxing, and soccer.

For what it's worth, hypnosis *is* still practiced in sports today, just not exactly in the way Tracy did it; it's more focused on self-hypnosis as opposed to the stage hypnosis that people tend to fear is mind control. One such modern-day practitioner, Ole Miss's assistant athletic director for sport psychology, Josie Nicholson, told me, "I always joke that when the siren goes off at twelve o'clock on Wednesdays you'll see a few athletes clucking like chickens, and that was me." Nicholson's generation of professionals was made possible by what was to come in the 1970s and 1980s.

* * *

Up to this point, my off-beat, selective summary of the history of sport psychology has been especially limited in a key dimension: Everyone I've discussed at length is a man. *Surely*, I thought while researching and writing, *there had to be influential women in the field. Maybe even women of color!* It's a no-brainer that they are changing the landscape of the industry in the present day and beyond, but I was 100 percent certain they must have also shaped sport psychology's past. It was a gap in my work that needed correcting, so I sought to do just that.

One of the people I spoke to in my effort to give women their due was Diane L. Gill, a professor in the kinesiology department at the University of North Carolina Greensboro. She had written in the history chapter of 2019's essential *Feminist Applied Sport Psychology*, edited by Leeja Carter, that "sport psychology has not embraced intersectionality and feminism but uncovering our feminist history may help develop the base to continue moving forward."[29] Despite gender bias, Gill told me, "women have always been there." She herself has been in the field since the 1970s, when it was largely still focused on physical education rather than psychology. She studied sport and exercise psychology. A couple of the bigger sport psychology organizations, the North American Society for the Psychology of Sport and Physical Activity and the Association for Applied Sport Psychology, both existed for about a decade before they had their first woman presidents. It's been only in the past 15 or 20 years, Gill told me, that psychology itself has become known as a female-dominated profession, including in academia.

"Women and women's issues have a place in sport psychology today, but too often that is an 'other' or special interest place," Gill wrote in 1995. "By taking steps to re-place women in history and by engendering current research and practice, sport and exercise psychology will be a stronger science and profession."[30]

I am not trying to make an all-inclusive list (who has the time or the pages?), but there are several people whose massive contributions to the field I find it particularly necessary to highlight and, like Gill said, help re-place in history. In the 1940s, Dorothy Hazeltine Yates was a psychology professor at what was then called San Jose State College. When teaching there, Kornspan said, athletes would often come up to her and ask whether she'd apply what she knew to help the college's sports programs. She apparently first declined but then relented and developed a relationship with the boxing team, which went undefeated while she was working with them, and later the track-and-field athletes. Athletes and aviators alike took her Psychology of Adjustment class, and many students in both categories would write to her years later to tell her how instrumental her class had been in their development (and, in some cases, their World War II experiences).

"[People] like to always say the 'fathers of,' right? And it's always fathers, right?" said Robin Vealey, a professor of sport psychology at Miami University (Ohio). "There's never any mothers. So the father of applied sport psychology was Bruce Ogilvie. Now, Bruce Ogilvie was amazing, and he did bridge the way for a lot of people. But why wouldn't we mention Dorothy Yates?"

A few decades later, in the 1970s, another Dorothy—Dorothy V. Harris—started a first-in-the-nation sport psychology graduate specialization at Penn State and also won the first Fulbright research scholarship in sport psychology. Harris was one of the first sport psychology residents at the Olympic Training Center, and her accolades only grew from there. Writing of Harris in 1992, one year after her death from pancreatic cancer, sport and exercise psychologist Deborah L. Feltz remembered, "She challenged me to be a creative thinker, to question assumptions, and to dig for the truth. She was an excellent role model for what women in sport psychology and in higher education could achieve."[31] Kornspan told me, "She doesn't get the credit that she probably should get."

I asked yet another key woman in the history of sport psychology, Carole Oglesby, what she thinks gets overlooked in her field. She quickly replied that things women did were seldom fully recognized. She is among those women, as other people I interviewed for this chapter have highlighted to me. Oglesby, a sport psychology emeritus professor and former Women's Sports Foundation trustee, has an "explicitly feminist voice [that] was often heard, although not so often welcomed, in sport psychology," Gill wrote of her breaking through in the 1970s.[32] In 1978, Oglesby edited the first book in the field, *Women and Sport: From Myth to Reality*, that featured what Gill described as a "clearly feminist perspective."

The three women above—Harris, Yates, and Oglesby—share something in common with the men featured heavily in this chapter: They are all white. Within the University of North Carolina Greensboro's kinesiology department, Gill, who is also white, estimated that she sees an equal mix of Black and white students alongside smaller but growing numbers of Latinx students. "It's getting closer to matching the athletes," Gill said, "being able to connect with the athletes, being able to see yourself. Representation matters. And that matters in academia, too."

Ruth Hall is another name that comes up again and again in these conversations about both gender and race in sport psychology. Hall, who is African American, takes an intersectional approach to the field. In a 2001 paper, she examined the role of race in both sports themselves and sport psychology. "How does feminist sport psychology relate to women of color?" Hall wrote. "First, feminism in and out of sport is still dominated in its thinking and writing by white, middle class, heterosexual women, most of whom assume that gender prevails as one's primary identification and, thus, minimizes the diversity within the feminist community." She went on to add that women of color are frequently viewed as "second-class citizens" in sport psychology. "More literature," she concluded, "is sorely needed."[33] I couldn't get a hold of Hall, who has retired from the College of New Jersey's psychology department, to discuss this in more detail, but I am willing to bet she'd say the same still unfortunately holds true more than two decades later.

* * *

Women and all, the true blossoming of sport psychology as a field was here at last in the latter half of the twentieth century. "Magically, sport psychology sort of appeared again in 1965," Kornspan said. "And obviously we knew that that actually didn't happen that way, right? I mean, there was stuff that was in the literature, but in a lot of our textbooks that's almost the way it was described, so people had this view that nothing occurred in sport psychology in the United States or even in the world before 1965." In reality, all the U.S. history we've reviewed, from Mosso to Griffith to Tracy, as well as history in countries like Russia, Germany, Japan, and later Brazil, Kornspan said, set the stage for the industry we know today. This increasing seriousness of the field was noted by leading sport psychologist Robert Singer in 1989: "The department that offered the graduate programs attempted to be academically rigorous and acceptable to other departments, to show that [sport psychology] was not merely a glorified 'jock' program, but rather a legitimate scientific area of study within sport sciences."[34]

The evolution of sports themselves also helped formalize and then revolutionize sport psychology. As teams in various men's sports moved out West and leagues expanded, players also started to recognize their value and unionize. They won the right to higher salaries, among other benefits, making them bigger investments for franchises. In the conclusion of *Psychology Gets in the Game*, Green and coeditor Ludy T. Benjamin sum up unionization's impact on sport psychology thusly: "Players became, more than ever before, expensive investments to be carefully nurtured. Their training and broader care increasingly required special expertise that traditional scouts and coaches could not offer—expertise such as that possessed by sport psychologists."[35]

The first journal dedicated exclusively to the field was the *International Journal of Sport Psychology*, founded in 1970. (The leading U.S. publication, the *Journal of Sport Psychology*, was still nine years away. Today, there are more than 35 English-language journals devoted to the field and closely related fields.)

In 1978, the U.S. Olympic Committee (now known as the U.S. Olympic and Paralympic Committee [USOPC]) created a sports medicine council that included sport psychologists. Four years later, the same committee created a registry of such professionals. And four years after *that*, the Association for Applied Sport Psychology was formed, becoming the largest such organization in the world. Around the same time, the American Psychological Association created Division 47, geared toward exercise and sport psychology. Early sport psychologists had training in exercise science and kinesiology, but in the 1980s, people trained as psychologists started entering the field in significant numbers, creating a turf war of sorts between the two factions. All were there, however, to help athletes feel and perform their best under pressure. So what does modern-day sport psychology look like in practice? It varies widely, but rest assured that no clucking chickens are involved.

CHAPTER 3

Science and Practice

What Mental Performance Coaches Actually Do

MENTAL PERFORMANCE COACHES ARE, YOU MIGHT SAY, ODDBALLS. IN one session that Paddy Steinfort later relayed to me, he insisted on saying, "Don't fuck this up," to a professional baseball player under his charge. He just kept repeating it. Also, "Don't hang the curveball. Don't hang it out there. I haven't got this pitch today. Is the coach coming out for a mound visit? Or is the GM in the stands looking at me right now?"[1]

These may not seem like constructive words, especially coming from a coach. They are, in fact, designed to push a player to their limits. Steinfort, a mental performance coach, is deliberately mimicking his athlete's own harsh internal monologue, as I detailed for *Sports Illustrated* in 2020. Hearing your own insecurities verbalized by someone else can be a frustrating and vulnerable experience, as he well knows. "I'll try and push your attention forward, I'll try and shift it to the dugout or to the stands," Steinfort told me then, "and your job as a performer is to bring it back to where I am right now."[2]

At the heart of it, the exercise Steinfort devised is about focusing on the task at hand—a conventional concept, just addressed in a bit of an unconventional way. He has worked with athletes across at least 10 sports, including professional basketball, football, baseball, swimming, rugby, soccer, golf, and even e-sports. He's also worked with the U.S. Army. His master's degree in applied psychology is from the University of Pennsylvania.

The kind of work that Steinfort—a six-foot-six Australian man who spent the first decade of his career as a ruckman in Aussie Rules—and others in the mental performance coaching profession do began at the elite level decades ago and is now finally becoming more common among all levels of sports.

Don Kalkstein, the Dallas Mavericks' longtime director of mental skills, said, "It's trickled its way down all the way, to some cases, into middle schools, and I could make the argument that it's in the primary school level, where they're teaching mindfulness training and simple meditation, which are mental skills as well." He believes that Mavs owner Mark Cuban and the franchise were the first in the NBA to employ someone in his role. Kalkstein landed the gig back in 2000 after a handful of years working with MLB's Texas Rangers, at which time he estimated there were just three or four other people in professional baseball providing that kind of training.

Jonathan F. Katz, a clinical and sport psychologist in Austin, Texas, who has worked in the field since 1990, described the early days as such: "The research was not very good," he said. "It was really all about underperformance. It's like [an athlete is] being sent to the principal's office." Katz, who has since worked with the NHL's New York Rangers, pro tennis players, and a host of other elite, college, and youth athletes, went on to clarify that he was happy to work with underperformers, but in those days, he especially craved the opportunity to work with people on the other end of the spectrum, those who were thriving. "I was always interested in the concept of the kid who's getting an A- or an A in class is being left alone and the kid who's getting the C's or D's gets the attention," he said. "The guys who were batting .310 and making the All-Star team, they get left alone. But don't they have a huge upside? Why aren't they batting .340?"

Sport psychology, Katz thought, was too reactive and not nearly proactive enough at the time, just like other areas of sports. "Athletes went to see the dietician if they were overweight," he said. "It was about seeing the trainer if you were injured." Katz recalled the season that Atlanta Braves right-handed pitcher John Smoltz started seeing a sport psychologist as one seminal moment in his field. Soon into Katz's career, after the

Smoltz news broke, he even started getting calls from people interested in finding jobs like his.

Smoltz, a future Cy Young winner with a Hall of Fame career ahead of him, carried a 2–11 record into the 1991 MLB All-Star break. He didn't exactly look like Cy Young material. But after the pause, he went 12–2 and wound up in the World Series with the Braves. So what had changed? During the break, Smoltz had consulted Jack Llewellyn, a former college pitcher who had worked with athletes since 1976. It was a move that people were clearly befuddled by at the time. "A good performance last night was going to make Dr. Jack the Sigmund Freud of the pastoral game," wrote Mike Littwin in the *Baltimore Sun*. "Traditionalists were prepared to be shocked. These are the guys who think the only worthwhile advance in the 20th century was the pop-top can."[3]

For all the jokes in the article, Littwin actually demystified sport psychology pretty effectively for a general audience coming in cold. He reported that the steps were simple: Llewellyn (who, by the way, was working with four other baseball teams at the time, too) got six hours of tape of Smoltz pitching and edited it down to two and a half minutes. The two analyzed the pitches together, and Llewellyn helped Smoltz pinpoint what he was doing right, mechanically and otherwise, and, perhaps even more important, how to *remember* what he was doing right and recover from bad pitches in the moment. "It's been a big key in my turnaround," Smoltz said at the time. "The main thing he taught me was to focus on the good and forget the bad."[4]

Llewellyn wasn't the only mental performance coach around in those days—not even the only one in baseball. There was Harvey Dorfman, sometimes known as the "godfather" of the sport's mental game. Starting in the mid-1980s with the Oakland Athletics, he collaborated behind the scenes with a slew of notable major leaguers, including Roy Halladay, Al Leiter, Greg Maddux, and Alex Rodriguez. Dorfman eventually left behind the team environment to work for mega-agent Scott Boras. His view of sport psychology work can be distilled down into one quip of his: "I'm not a shrink—I'm a stretch."[5] Like Llewellyn, he was there to pinpoint what was off in a player's performance—what might be holding him back mentally—and help him develop a plan to course-correct.

(Dorfman died in 2011, leaving behind a host of wonderful and influential books, including a two-part autobiography.)

Outside of baseball, Briana Scurry is another prominent athlete who made use of a sport psychologist in the 1990s. The goalkeeper for the U.S. women's national soccer team knew she had to get any edge possible to retain her starting spot. "[My father] was always someone that said, 'Bri, you can always learn something new.' And so when [mental skills coach Colleen] Hacker came along, some people thought she had her voodoo and her woo-woo psychology. It was all new back then. It wasn't like the industry it is now," Scurry said in 2022. "She was a pioneer in what she was doing."

In net, Scurry said she would get frustrated when she was scored on. It's only natural in a position where one mistake can do enough damage to knock the team out of a World Cup. Hacker helped her compartmentalize. "She said, 'Bri, I want you to try this. When you give up a goal, you have between the time when that goal is scored and the kickoff to dwell on it and to be upset about it, and then what I want you to do, once the whistle blows, you put it in the package and you put it on the shelf. It'll be there. We have the game footage. We can look at it later,'" Scurry recalled. "And that one thing revolutionized my goalkeeping."

Athletes of Smoltz's and Scurry's caliber almost definitely worked way harder to transform and sustain their decorated careers than they let on. From their examples, sport psychology sounds so easy to teach and learn, but there's an art and science to it that are far more complicated than an average fan might assume.

* * *

Remember the days of Coleman Roberts Griffith, flailing with the Chicago Cubs? Sport psychology has needed decades since then—and plenty of open-minded athletes like Smoltz and Scurry—to take off, but now it's soaring. Many colleges, pro leagues, teams, and national governing bodies employ sport psychologists and mental performance coaches. While it might sound like there's a simple—if intangible—formula for success (using charm and character to nudge players into sharing their feelings and sharpening their performances), the reality is much more rooted in complex scientific and creative techniques. But every athlete, even those on the same team, requires a unique approach when it comes to everything from the squishy concept of mindfulness to the somehow even squishier concept of mental toughness.

Neha Uberoi, a former professional tennis player (once ranked as high as world No. 196 in singles) and current psychotherapist working at Valera Health, a tele-behavioral health platform, takes a somewhat sneaky approach to her work with athletes. "Sometimes the only way in as a clinician is through their performance," said Uberoi, who also heads up the networking group South Asians in Sports and works in mental performance coaching with athletes. "'I don't want to come in here and have you tell me there's an issue,'" she said, describing what some clients tell her. "'I just want you to help me be a better athlete.' That's often an avenue for obsessive-compulsive behavioral thoughts or intrusive thoughts. When you tie it back to the performance piece, the athlete is more likely to be receptive."

So how do top-tier athletes become mentally tough, mindful, and all those other supposedly good things? Their various athletic coaches and trainers help, sure, but they also, increasingly, turn to mental performance experts like the ones we've met so far. "Sixty years ago, the head coach did everything. They were the technical coach, they were the physical coach, they were the mental coach, they were the life coach, they were the nutritionist. They did it all," said Michael Gervais, the high-performance coach. He's been in the business for about 30 years and has seen it explode firsthand. "And then the emerging science of strength and conditioning came online, and the progressive coaches back then said, 'Wait a minute, I don't know if I'm gonna trust these people, these strength and conditioning people. But if we are bigger, faster, stronger in the fourth quarter, wow, that'd be great.' So they started to bring them on. . . . Then there was a cascade and a copycat experience across other coaches and leagues. And then those same coaches, those avant-garde coaches, were like, 'Wait, what's that? You know what? These guys are bigger, faster, stronger. We need better medical.' So the [athletic training and physical therapy] world started to explode inside of clubs. Then came nutrition.

Then, once you've got physical, you've got the medical, and you've got nutrition, what's next? Psychology."

About 25 years ago, in Gervais's estimation, it was the "explorers" (the more adventurous team coaches or managers) seeking out mental performance coaches, most of whom were also researchers and professors at universities because there was little to no full-time work to be had in sport psychology. About 10 years ago, he really noticed the field taking off, with many Seattle Seahawks players he worked with having come from colleges that used such professionals.

Seeing a mental skills or performance coach is not necessarily equivalent to seeing a clinical psychologist or social worker for mental health counseling. The former titles do not require the provider to be a licensed therapist (though some such coaches do also have doctorates or other forms of specialization in clinical psychology). Neither are they licensed psychiatrists. So if they encounter any clinical issues, like depression or generalized anxiety disorder, for example, in the course of mental performance coaching, they have to refer the athlete out to a provider with the proper credentials. On the distinction between mental performance coaches and clinicians who work with athletes, a couple of schools of thought exist: Some experts see professionals in mental performance coaching as being potentially helpful to athletes' performance, while others believe athletes should meet with only licensed psychologists, social workers, and psychiatrists.

Steven C. Hayes, a clinical psychologist and a professor of behavioral health at the University of Nevada, Reno, told me he falls more or less into the first camp. "All of this training can actually make it systematically impossible to talk to normal people," he argued. "I'm not impressed by the letters that come after someone's name independently of their proven ability to make a difference in athletes' lives in a way that develops and sustains not just athletic performance but the whole person."

Ideally, Hayes said, he wants someone to have the capacity to read and internalize the relevant scientific literature in sport psychology but also be a "real person" who can communicate with athletes on their level—"to not have been socialized in the *psychobabble blah blah blah* that actually only intimidates and makes people around you feel less connected to you." He did warn, though, that mental performance coaches who are not psychologists by trade are more susceptible to "lay ideas" that may have worked for one athlete once but may not apply by and large to elite performers.

Uberoi, on the other hand, said she falls into the second camp: She thinks that anyone working with athletes should have a strong clinical background. "The person who's just coming in and wondering about mental performance doesn't understand what could go wrong," she said. "There are a lot of techniques and words and signs that you're not looking for that can lead an athlete into a worse situation."

She took her train of thought a step further, too, explaining that she believes that every professional who works with athletes should have a background in sports themselves. "We forget what it's actually like to be out there," she said. "I respect someone a lot more who's gone through it rather than someone who's just only been an academic." Chris Carr, the Green Bay Packers' director of performance psychology and behavioral health clinician, also noted that you can't just pick up an issue of *Sports Illustrated* or coach your kid's tee-ball team as a psychologist and declare yourself a *sport* psychologist. Specific experience in athletics, he said, does matter. Katz feels similarly. "Some psychologists who gave a motivational talk to their eight-year-old's soccer team put on their bio that they do sport psychology," Katz said. "It's buyer beware."

There are so many support staffers around athletes nowadays that you can't really blame them if they are not able to tell who's who anymore, credential-wise. Kalkstein, for example, used to get people resisting the idea of meeting with him because they were thinking they didn't want to lay down in his office, like they might in a stereotypical shrink's office, and focus solely on recounting and processing their childhood trauma. "While [clinical psychologists] are extremely important and do play a role in performance, we are really focusing more on performance issues," he said, such as, in Steinfort's example, how to stay zeroed in on throwing your best pitches without getting distracted by internal or external factors.

The requirements, degrees, and certificates for working with athletes also vary widely both nationally and internationally. Daria Abramowicz, a sport and performance psychologist in Poland, described to me the lack of regulation in her country. "Basically, in Poland, if you read some books and if you think, *Hmm, I am a good listener and I am good with talking to people*, and then you put the plate on your door like you're a mental coach, you're fine," she said disapprovingly. "No one will penalize you for that." Abramowicz has been in the field about a decade, following a career in sailing. She works with renowned tennis player Iga Świątek, who's been ranked world No. 1, and 15 or 20 other athletes.

In reality, the sport psychology profession is fluid and complex, and despite the varying and sometimes lacking requirements, these aren't skills that just anyone can master. There's a whole evolving science behind the field, Hayes has told me in conversations for *Sports Illustrated* and this book. You can often demonstrate that a mental performance coach has done a good job, with actual, measurable evidence. "[Sport psychology] requires practice," he said in 2020. "This is not woo-woo. You can show it at the physiological . . . level."[6]

* * *

Sport psychology, Hayes believes, has been moving away from a "one-size-fits-all model, into a more individual model." It goes back to the concept he mentioned about the dangers of thinking that a "lay idea" that worked for one athlete could work for all. That might seem obvious, but the field is still catching up to that reality.

Here, Hayes used an example of placing someone in front of a building and telling them they have to get to the other side. So the person goes through the front door into the vestibule, and immediately they're met with another glass door. That second one's locked. There are, however, doors down to the basement and up to the fire escape. Of course, the person could also leave the building and walk around the left or right side. If you think about how many people individually handled this situation, the averaged data would tell you to walk straight ahead. "Everyone's going to bust their face into the glass door if they do that," Hayes said. It's a good reminder that what works on average or in the aggregate means nothing for distinct, individual people—in this case elite athletes.

This newer approach to sport psychology takes the emphasis off that faux wisdom ("walk through the glass door") in favor of what the science shows. "How do you actually measure psychological skills in a way that's idiographic and fits the person?" Hayes asked. "It gives you concepts that you can apply to other people but doesn't homogenize people into the average that tells you to run through the closed glass door instead of: What are the unique ways you can get from here to there?"

As I noted in *Sports Illustrated* in 2020, Hayes offered the following example when explaining the scientific quality of mental performance coaching: A 2018 *Frontiers in Psychology* study of elite-level hockey players in Sweden showed that a high flexibility, or mindfulness, score is correlated to an increase in players' assists and a team's points. (A flexibility score is measured by an adaptation of a common psychological questionnaire.)

Hayes also pointed to the Stroop test. That's a neuropsychological experiment you're probably familiar with: The word "blue" might be written on the screen in the color green. The test taker is then asked to supply the color of the word rather than how it reads. It's not so easy, but focused athletes quickly arrive at the correct answer, Hayes said. How does that translate to sports, then? As I wrote for *Sports Illustrated*, mindfulness is a tool that allows players to adapt to situational changes. It can help them process what's happening at the peripheries of their vision. That's how they might be able to predict where their teammates are on the court.

The point of all this—the Stroop test, mindfulness scores, other exercises—is not to turn athletes into people they aren't. "I don't think you're necessarily trying to produce monks or create some great transformational spiritual experience," Hayes told me. "You're trying to help people be centered in the moment and help allocate their attention in a flexible, fluid, and voluntary way with all of the various things that are going to happen." He said the idea is to ultimately make them more mindful, focused, and successful.

So how does one make athletes more focused, fluid, and flexible performers? Steinfort's exercise to start the chapter is one untraditional way. It's one tiny bit of a four-pronged approach he uses to coach athletes through mental performance issues. First comes mindfulness, which he also calls awareness. This involves an athlete's acceptance of both external and internal realities. On the field, someone might say to themselves, "I don't feel good right now, but I don't need to feel perfect to execute this next thing." The second part is accepting the truth: that they aren't perfect. Third is committing to using a set of behaviors and intentional strategies, Steinfort said. (He related this to my profession by walking me through what I need to do to execute a good journalistic interview. I have to do research beforehand, ask good questions, follow up on the interviewee's answers, and stay attuned to their emotions throughout.) The fourth part is where Steinfort's work shines the most: teaching self-reflection that's both critical and accurate. It's asking yourself why you may not have executed the plan for a great interview or, in Steinfort's initial exercise, a transcendent, dialed-in performance on the mound. "How did I handle [a distraction], and how can I do it better?" Steinfort said athletes must ask themselves. He helps them find the answers.

All these steps are, in a way, meant to remind athletes that they are, in fact, performers. And performance requires practice, not just on the physical level but on the mental one, too. "Just like you're going to be practicing forehands and backhands, if you're not meditating and doing visualization techniques and strengthening your mind to be able to per-form," you won't achieve the results you're looking for, Uberoi said. "It is a muscle. It can be trained. If you're not working on it along with all the other stuff you're doing physically, it's going to be very hard for you to succeed."

* * *

Before tennis matches, the Romanian Canadian player Bianca Andreescu routinely does visualization and mindfulness exercises. "At first I was like, what is this bullshit?" the one-time U.S. Open champion told me. "And then I saw that it was working." It all goes back to her childhood, when she said she had the "worst temper" on the court. When she was 13 or 14, her mom decided it was time for her to learn how to visualize—some-thing, anything, to calm down a bit and hopefully stop breaking essential equipment. "I'm done paying for more rackets," Andreescu remembered her mother saying.

The process started out slowly. Every day, she'd spend two minutes on mindfulness, regulating her breathing, then five, 10, and 15 minutes and soon a full hour (much longer than she does on a regular basis now). "I was becoming more calm," Andreescu told me. "I was becoming more happy on the court, even if I was losing." Andreescu also developed an exercise where she would write something negative and throw the piece of paper away (e.g., "I feel like shit"). Then she would write down a win of the day to keep. "I kept my composure," or maybe "I read 30 minutes of a book," or "if it was a big thing—I won the U.S. Open—even better," she explained, laughing.

There's a famous story that goes around about Andreescu's history of visualization. When she was 15 or 16, she wrote herself a fake check for the U.S. Open prize money. She dated it—you guessed it—2019, the year she beat Serena Williams in the final. "It just shows you the power of manifestation," she stressed to me.

For another elite athlete, two-time Paralympic triathlete silver medalist and two-time world champion Hailey Danz, mental health and mental performance are "a topic in every conversation" that she has with her teammates. She started seeing a sport psychologist affiliated with the USOPC in the months leading up to the 2016 Rio Games. The development proved major when, after the Olympics, she experienced a difficult comedown. ("I wouldn't say I was clinically depressed, but I think that I had that mild, constant little buzz of something," is how she put it to me five years later.)

Danz continued seeing a sport psychologist regularly post-Rio, working primarily on mindfulness. "In triathlon, there's so much going on," she said. "It's a long time to be out there with your thoughts. My race is an hour and 15 minutes. It's not a 100-meter dash where you can just have one cue and think about that the entire time." She began to feel more self-aware, more focused. After Tokyo in 2021, thanks to her added focus on mental performance, she had no major issues with the post-Games comedown.

CHAPTER 3

Paralympians face extra sets of challenges compared with even other elite athletes, Danz said. First, there's the matter of classification that weighs on many of them. Paralympic sports are organized into classes that separate competitors by degree of "severity" of their disabilities. There have been well-documented stories of athletes' potentially cheating to move up in classification to compete against athletes who may not be in their same true class and thus have an easier time beating their opponents. "If you spend any amount of time with any para-athlete, this is going to come up," Danz said. "'This person should be in this class but they're in this class, and I'm not winning this because they're in the wrong class.' I feel like it really does wear on people's mental health." The discussion is so pervasive that she and her teammates implemented a rule that they can't discuss classification.

Another issue unique to Paralympians and other disabled athletes is the high cost of necessary adaptive equipment. Danz needs $10,000 bikes to compete and $20,000 running legs (she is a left-leg amputee). Those are paid for mostly with her funding from the national team, but up-and-coming athletes don't have access to such money and a living stipend. Similarly, athletes who use wheelchairs need expensive racing chairs. Blind athletes have to pay for not only themselves to get into races, but also their guides. "Everybody has something," said Chris Murphy, a Paralympic cyclist for the United States. He used to serve on the USOPC's mental health task force. "With Paralympians, it's pretty much a given that we all have something that we're dealing with. That's more or less the criteria of being a Paralympian." He laughed. All of this is to say that athletes are up against all sorts of challenges that influence their mental health and mental performance, varying by sport, ability level, country, age, and many other factors.

* * *

Carrie Carpenter, who has worked with the St. Louis Cardinals for many years as well as with the Dallas Mavericks and Southern Methodist University, said a lot of her job is triage. There's pressure. "You feel like you're in an emergency room with them and if you don't tell them this

50

golden piece of advice right then, if they don't go out and fix it, will they ever come back [to my office]?" she said. Mental performance, she must remind her athletes, is not a "magic pill."

Past the triage point, sport psychologists and mental performance coaches have the opportunity to get creative—really creative—to keep athletes coming back. Steinfort speaks the athlete's internal monologue aloud. Abramowicz often scours a local bookstore's games section. Nothing is off limits for her work: board games, card games, drawing tools, even Lego bricks.

"There are a lot of exercises that are improving cognitive abilities, such as focus, attention, solving problems, analytical thinking, hand–eye coordination, sometimes working with the nervous system," she said. "That's why I work really closely with strength and conditioning coaches, so we have full system control." So how does Lego factor in for athletes? Abramowicz excitedly showed me one Lego build in her apartment over Zoom. (Full disclosure: I own a Lego typewriter. No, it isn't fully functional. No ink.) She explained that Lego is not only fun; it's also meant to enhance cognitive abilities. Building-block activities require skills like focus, analytical thinking, motor control, and hand–eye coordination.

One of Carpenter's favorite tactics is similarly simple. She knows that performance coaching is all about building relationships. "Asking them how they're doing. Asking how their family is doing," she said. "Do you need anything from me? Just stuff like that. It's laid-back, very casual." In working with athletes who are often experiencing anxiety, Carpenter wants to "give them their power back." "I always tell them that your anxiety is a monster. Your emotions feed the monster, but your thoughts starve it, right? So if we can think clearly and we can think well, that's the way to keep the anxiety at bay and get back to who you are and what you love doing."

To foster trust and get to know a professional or collegiate athlete, a common exercise Carpenter uses is asking them, on a scale from 1 to 10, where their "sweet spot" is when performing. One is "super chill," and 10 is "really amped up." Someone may compete their best at a 4, others a 6 or 7. The athletes begin to visualize and describe in detail what their ideal setting looks like. Over time and close work with Carpenter, the athletes truly begin to "own" their numbers, she said, becoming experts at snapping into their ideal performance state.

Despite the creative techniques Steinfort employs, he is careful to say that despite the snapshots of the job he might showcase on platforms like Instagram, a lot of the work is more rote. "Some people think I'm just there talking about the pressure of a free throw when in reality it could be the mundanity of 'Did you do that stretching program you were supposed to do this morning?'" he said. "'Did you meditate properly? What was your experience when you meditated?'"

A key part of that work with athletes is meeting them where they're at when coming up with exercises and explaining their benefits. No one's likely to meditate if they can't understand why they're doing it in the first place. That's where Ben Freakley's work has been groundbreaking. The sport and performance psychology coach, who has a specialization in clinical mental health (at a non-doctorate level), followed in Steinfort's footsteps by working with MLB's Toronto Blue Jays, eventually heading up a performance department of as many as six people. He wanted a way to communicate with athletes on their own level.

So Freakley created a book called *The Separator*, all about mental performance techniques pulled from core tenets of Hayes's ideology but translated into more accessible language. (For example, he changed a principle called "cognitive defusion," part of acceptance and commitment therapy, to the much more easily comprehensible "thoughts aren't facts." Cognitive defusion is the process of realizing that our thoughts aren't literally true.) The book is available in both English and Spanish, an offering Freakley is hugely proud of given the number of Latino players working in the team's system and throughout baseball.

In five chapters of a slim volume, *The Separator* combines Hayes's ideology with elements of positive psychology, like instructing players to remind themselves of their strengths instead of just overanalyzing their weaknesses. Throughout the book, Freakley, who played Division I soccer as a forward at Georgia Southern, and his colleagues (both within the mental performance department and across other departments) sprinkled in relevant success stories of pro athletes as well as artists and military personnel. "We just asked ourselves, 'What would you want to read about if you were in [the players'] shoes?'" Freakley said. "So we kept it short, we tried to keep it interesting, and we wanted to make it really actionable."

Neither Freakley nor I have heard of any other professional sports organizations creating such a handbook for players and coaches to use. (When I asked for a copy of the book, I was met with the polite reply, "That's just for the Jays.") Yes, coaches, too—he pointed out that those who work most closely with players around success and failure should be equipped with the same tools the players are. When I asked whether Freakley had a sense of how widely read *The Separator* was or is, he said he didn't know for sure. But he emphasized that it's clearly had some sort of impact because some of the ideas mentioned in the book have become "tribal language" throughout the organization.

As for a specific exercise Freakley thinks resonates well with players, he recalled a time when he visited the Blue Jays' Triple-A affiliate. Almost every player was in attendance. He had each guy hold three baseballs in one hand as he led an awareness-of-breath exercise, or mindfulness meditation. As Freakley guided them, he'd have each drop one baseball and then a second one, until one baseball was left. Then he'd have them squeeze the remaining baseball super tightly.

"The best links are when they link something that we do onto how it relates to their own performance on the field," Freakley said. "And so the conclusion that they did get to was that one of the baseballs represents the past, one of the baseballs represents the future, and how much more energy we can focus on the present when we have a willingness to let go of what has happened—that's the acceptance piece in all of this—and also when we have a willingness to notice when our mind is really worried about the future, and we let go of that as well. Then we can regulate our attention back onto the present moment."

* * *

Freakley said that he considers mental performance training to be about far more than one-on-one work with an athlete. It's about getting teammates together, like he did with the breathing exercise we just walked through, and letting them discuss approaches and draw their own conclusions. It's also about staying out and about with the athletes, an idea I've heard echoed by many of the professionals I spoke with: "I think you're going to get a lot more buy-in building relationships being around fields and competitions, as opposed to being in an office," Freakley said.

Increasingly, his predecessor with the Blue Jays, Steinfort, is finding himself working more frequently with one athlete at a time, apart from his gig with the Australian men's and women's national soccer teams. It's a shift he described as organic now that the Australian native has more experience both in the field and living in the United States. Individual athletes in various leagues are approaching him, sometimes through their agents or sometimes through their own connections with Steinfort from previous teams they played for. Maybe a certain athlete's current team doesn't provide a mental performance coach, or maybe the athlete just doesn't jibe with the professional on hand. It's similar to how an elite NBA player might find independent shooting coaches or physical therapists to up their game.

The connection between the mental performance coach and the athlete is critical, Steinfort said. "If the player doesn't trust you, it's very hard to get an authentic account of their actual experience and get them to be honest about, 'I was scared in this moment.'" An example: Steinfort recalled a specific "come to Jesus" call with an NBA player early in the season. With the athlete, he referred back to a preseason conversation about what he called the basketball player's three main emotional opponents: anxiety, anger, and apathy. Steinfort asked the athlete whether any of those three had shown up in the past couple of weeks, a rough patch for him. He responded, "Dude, just in the last three days, I've had all three of them." That admission requires a level of trust that needs to develop organically, or progress tackling those opponents can't be made.

Steinfort also pointed out that athletes can find mental performance coaches just about anywhere today; it's as simple as scrolling through Instagram or TikTok. "If a coach or someone markets themselves very well and puts their stuff out there and they're legit—or let's be honest, even if they're not legit but they market themselves well—there is more access for individuals to find their own providers," Steinfort said. "Back when I was an athlete, if I wanted to find a psychologist, I had to buy a book and look in the back of it to find their landline phone number and ring them to see if they will do a session." (While that proliferation of experts and people posing as experts can be dangerous, Steinfort noted that most elite athletes have great "bullshit radars.")

Confidentiality is one key factor athletes must weigh when deciding whether to see a mental performance coach provided by their team. A lot of athletes choose to work with independent professionals like Steinfort because they like the clear degree of separation he has from the team. He doesn't report to the coach, the general manager, or the owner.

For athletes working with team providers, "It may be very hard for that individual to be fully honest with you and then wonder, *Is that going to go to the head coach? Who might go, He's not supposed to be angry at me for doing this or he's not supposed to have anxiety when he's shooting free throws*," Steinfort said. How will the guy working extensively with the performance coach get treated when his contract is up? And, as Steinfort brought up to me, will team officials view someone as less reliable if there's an admission of mental illness—or even just performance-related struggles? "That is a real stigma that exists in the world in general and definitely still impacts performers," he said. "So they need to be cautious who they let into those very intimate conversations."

* * *

When I was reporting this chapter, one part of my conversation with Steinfort caught me a bit off guard. In one of my first questions to him in our chat just before Thanksgiving of 2022, I accidentally suggested that mental performance and mental health were two totally discrete concepts, and he called me on it. I'm glad he did. For the purposes of this book, I often use those two terms to make distinctions—the mind's role in on-field (or on-court) performance versus the mental illness that crops up and affects people on the field and off.

But those terms don't represent a dichotomy, Steinfort argued—and I agreed. He brought up the famous example of Simone Biles (whom we'll discuss in more detail in chapter 6) taking a step back from most Olympic events in 2021 when she was having trouble landing skills on her feet. "There's still very simplistic thinking in the sense of, *Oh, Simone pulled out because she wasn't mentally able to do it*," Steinfort said, suggesting our vocabulary typically isn't precise enough to handle the nuance of these situations. "Does that mean it's a mental health episode, or has she lost her ability to orient in space?"

Steinfort is saying that, to the best of his knowledge, he believes Biles's struggles at those Olympics started out as the latter—a *performance* issue, not an *illness* one. It's, as Steinfort said, a "mixed picture," in his mind, because her performance issues very well might have led to issues more traditionally classified as mental illness. (Only Biles and those who have treated her know for sure.)

Carr has a similar view of mental performance and mental health, saying that they fall on a continuum. "It's not, 'Are we doing mental training or doing mental health?'" he said. "In my role, all of performance psychology is about mental health." That reminded me of Hayes's philosophy as well. He likes to say, referring to the popular statistic that one in five adults is affected by mental illness, that mental health is not a one-in-five issue, it's a five-in-five issue. "We all need to work on our mental strength and flexibility the same way that we need to work on our physical strength and flexibility," he said. "If you're not exercising, you're not doing some weightlifting, you're not doing some cardio, you're not doing some stretching exercises, what the hell are you doing?"

I asked LaTisha Bader, a licensed psychologist, certified mental performance consultant, and licensed addiction counselor who works for the Denver-based, gender-specific intensive outpatient program Women's Recovery, whether it's possible to fully tease out mental performance from mental health. She immediately said no: "They're just so intertwined."

As we shift our focus in the coming chapters largely to the mental illness side of the spectrum, it's important to remember that all players can benefit from working on their minds and that it's a good idea to seek help in that area *before* there's a problem to speak of. And that goes for us normies, too, not just elite athletes: "We have our own mental performance challenges, and maybe they're not world-class, but they're challenging us," Hayes said. "So it's going home and talking to your loved one or getting to work and really giving it your all or whatever. Five out of five, 24/7."

PART II

THE MEGAPHONE

Speaking Out about Mental Illness

CHAPTER 4

The Firsts

Trailblazers Who Came Forward

BEFORE IT WAS EVEN SOMEWHAT SOCIALLY ACCEPTABLE TO SPEAK UP about mental illness, even before many players were vocal about working with mental performance coaches, there were a few athletes willing to risk their careers to make their voices heard. Prominent athlete pioneers moved the ball steadily forward, essentially daring people to keep ignoring the health and livelihood of the performers they idolize in favor of fawning over their athletic pursuits.

There were many such athletes struggling in eras when speaking up about mental illness was taboo.[1] Here, we'll highlight a few relatively recent figures, imperfections and all, who took risks in coming forward: Chamique Holdsclaw, Pete Harnisch, Bill Pulsipher, Royce White, and—finally—Michael Phelps. They took those risks not necessarily because they wanted to but because they had to. In that sense, lifting up these athletes is a bit of an awkward thing: It's not the kind of spotlight they sought out for their athletic achievements. It's not even attention they necessarily earned in any way. But here we are, and here these athletes were.

Holdsclaw was a world-class athlete, a standout basketball player who had won three consecutive NCAA championships with Tennessee. She had also been the first pick in the 1999 WNBA draft. As she grew older, she realized that in one key way, she had no role models in her sport—or any sport. Rather, Catherine Zeta-Jones was her North Star. It may seem like a strange comparison for an athlete to make to an actor, but Zeta-Jones was the only famous person Holdsclaw knew in the early 2010s who had been open about having bipolar disorder. "Her name kept coming up," Holdsclaw said, "and I'm like, *Wow, man, this lady is so amazing, so successful, and she's able to share this and move forward in her life. She can do it, I can do it also.*" They even had the same kind: type II, which is characterized by long periods of depression and shorter bursts of hypomania. The latter typically entails an elevated mood and emotions (essentially, a shorter, less severe form of the mania that accompanies bipolar I).

Holdsclaw's lows had been quite low. In the summer of 2004, while with the Washington Mystics, she didn't show up for a game. The star locked herself in her town house with all the lights off, not even opening up the door for Pat Summitt, who was the Mystics' player personnel consultant, her legendary college coach, and a mother figure of hers. This was just two years after Holdsclaw's grandmother, June, who had raised her since age 11 in Astoria, Queens, had died. In fact, Holdsclaw ended up stepping away for the rest of the season. She shut down, even changing her cell phone number to avoid Summitt.

Months after that skipped game and shortened season, Holdsclaw came out about her experience with depression, her diagnosis at the time, in an interview with the *Washington Post*'s Sally Jenkins, clearing up the "undisclosed medical reasons" cited at the time she stepped away. "Everything was negative," she told Jenkins. "Dark." The pressure of being an elite athlete had gotten to her, as we now know. "I just didn't want to be Chamique," she added. "People look at me, even my family and friends, in an almost supernatural way. I just wanted to be a regular person."[2]

Her circumstances were still getting darker, too. In 2006, she attempted suicide during her time with the Los Angeles Sparks. "I felt I had no control, and it was a constant struggle. I said, 'Hey, I'm successful, I'm in control on the court and able to do these great things,'" Holdsclaw would later say of the suicide attempt. "But when it came to issues of the mind, I couldn't get a grip on it."[3]

The only place where Holdsclaw's troubles didn't get in her way was indeed on the court. "I love my sport," she told me in 2022. "I'm locked in. I'm focused. I'm doing something that I enjoy, and that's when I would say my mind wasn't working against me. It was endorphins. Everything was hitting at once. That was my peace." At home, away from the sport, the "crafty little creature on [her] shoulder" would turn dark for her, she added.

Back in June of the 2007 season, the year after her suicide attempt, Holdsclaw stunned the Los Angeles Sparks and the league when she abruptly announced her retirement. "This was not an easy decision," she said in a team statement.[4] Later that month, she elaborated a bit to the *Los Angeles Times*, saying, "I made my decision because I just didn't feel it anymore. It was like, 'This is it.'" Holdsclaw wanted people to know that she stepped away from the game due to her lack of interest as well as her desire to spend time with family and friends—not her mental illness: "Let people know I'm not depressed."[5]

Holdsclaw returned to the WNBA in 2009, after her rights had been traded the previous winter to the Atlanta Dream. "It's not about me anymore," she said then. "I've always been a player who just played. I have to use my voice a little more now, give back to young people dealing with the problems I've had." The *New York Times* write-up of her comeback, like much of journalism on mental health in sports, left a lot to be desired: "With her illness in check and her game in tow, Holdsclaw ended her hiatus this year, driven to show others afflicted by depression that it is beatable."[6] That's one inspiring way to frame it, but it wouldn't be the end of the star's story with mental illness.

For the second and final time, Holdsclaw stepped away from the WNBA, after the 2010 season. Three years later, she pleaded guilty to two counts of aggravated assault, possession of a firearm during the commission of a felony, criminal damage in the first degree, and two counts of criminal damage in the second degree. The charges stemmed from an incident that had occurred in 2012, when Holdsclaw broke an ex-girlfriend's Range Rover's windows with a bat and fired a shot into the SUV. (No one was injured.) She was sentenced to three years' probation and a $3,000 fine. Of the crime, Holdsclaw said at the time, "It was real uncharacteristic of me."

After years of being misdiagnosed as having just depression (a common experience, shared by yours truly), Holdsclaw, after the guilty plea, may have been one of the first athletes with her level of fame to step forward and say she's bipolar. Through her attorneys, Holdsclaw had worked with a forensic psychologist who reviewed a decade of her medical records and determined that bipolar II was an accurate diagnosis. "I was angry," Holdsclaw said. "I'm like, 'Come on.' I've been going through this pretty much since I was a young kid. I've been on medications trying different things since 2002, and you tell me it takes a situation like this for people to really look at it and get the right medications." (Perhaps this is a good place for a reminder that mentally ill people are more likely to be victims of violent crimes than perpetrators of them.)

Now, as Holdsclaw raises young kids with her wife, new generations of athletes routinely approach her to tell her about their struggles with mental illness and seek advice. It's something the Hall of Famer couldn't have pictured back when she was struggling without an accurate label to point to or peers to commiserate with, but she's learned to be more vulnerable in the years since her retirement.

"I had this wall up to protect myself from the media, and I finally just had to say, you know what? Look in the mirror, and you know I'm not perfect, let this wall down, start to have these conversations and tell people how I feel," she told me. "If someone's hurt me, say something to address it because I would keep a lot of stuff inside, and eventually, like I always say, if there's a bag and you keep stuffing it and stuffing it and stuffing it, eventually it's gonna spill out."

When athletes were going through hard times, they often didn't have supportive teammates, coaches, or staff to turn to—or at the very least, due to stigma and a lack of education about available resources, they didn't *think* they did. Back at Tennessee in the 1990s, Holdsclaw declined to meet with the sport psychologist, fearing what would happen if others in her program saw her working with one. "I'm the captain. I'm the leader of the team. They're gonna think that I'm weak," Holdsclaw said, reflecting back on her mindset at the time.

It wasn't until the end of Holdsclaw's professional career, in 2010, when she was with the San Antonio Silver Stars (now the Las Vegas

Aces), that she directly filled in a coach on her mental illness. It was also around that time, in either 2009 or 2010, Holdsclaw recalled, that on the first day of training camp, coaches put up on a board resources for doctors and mental health professionals. She reasoned that she may have been more open earlier had previous teams of hers taken that simple step.

* * *

In 1997, two years before Holdsclaw was drafted into the WNBA, Pete Harnisch, a veteran right-handed pitcher for the New York Mets, unexpectedly left his team. It seemed no one knew exactly why. He was on the injured (then called "disabled") list. A *New York Times* headline called him "troubled" and reported that the Mets were themselves still unsure of the reason for Harnisch's absence, though he had been put through physical and psychological testing. Harnisch had quit chewing tobacco the month before—maybe he was feeling withdrawal symptoms? There was also speculation that he had a recurrence of Lyme disease or simply a loss of confidence.

Twenty days went by before Harnisch said anything. In a 20-minute press conference call, he announced, "I'd just like to let everybody know I've been diagnosed with depression."

"I felt very withdrawn," Harnisch said. "I felt very much to myself." The 30-year-old nine-year veteran was in therapy and taking medicine, he told journalists that spring day. He also briefly acknowledged a family history of depression. Harnisch's disclosure came years before MLB would even enact policies specifying disabled list/injured list placement for mental health reasons.

In 1997, we were still a decade away from something like the outcry over Britney Spears's head-shaving incident and the barbaric, mental illness–related shaming. (It still follows her to this day.) Harnisch likely felt his environment was a hostile one to be speaking up in.

The pitcher's initial statement was so significant to Bowling Green communication professor Raymond I. Schuck that he wrote a chapter in the 2019 book *Sport, Rhetoric, and Political Struggle* centered on its significance. It was fittingly titled, highlighting Harnisch's own words, "'I'd

Just Like to Let Everybody Know': Pete Harnisch on the Disabled List
and the Politics of Mental Health." (Side note: I got to this chapter from
Mike Delayo, the Penn State graduate student researching the rhetoric of
popular culture through sport, and his excellent thesis on mental health
disclosure in professional sports. His thesis is *also* perfectly titled: "I
Definitely Want to Thank My Psychiatrist," in a nod to basketball great
Metta Sandiford-Artest.)

In Schuck's view, Harnisch's disclosure was big. "Harnisch's admission . . . advanced discourse on mental health by offering public acknowl-
edgement of his condition and thereby designating the legitimacy of
mental health, at least in the form of depression, reason for [disabled list]
placement," Schuck wrote. He also noted that Harnisch's listing to the
press of symptoms, including anxiety, loss of appetite, and weight loss,
helped, too, by painting a clear picture of what he was going through.

At the same time, Schuck argued, Harnisch's statement also may
have held back progress a bit (he makes clear to say he's not personally
criticizing the baseball player). "His description of symptoms located the
condition within himself as an individual without indication of structural
conditions of working in sport that may have contributed to them," he
wrote. It's a tall order, as Schuck seems to realize, for one person—especially around that time, before the majority of us were sensitive to such
disclosures from famous people—to address not only their own personal
condition mere weeks after receiving a diagnosis, but also the systemic
factors in play that make sports an environment that could foster mental
illness.

As time went on, Harnisch would say more about his depression.
When he first started experiencing it in March 1997, he was unable to
sleep more than an hour or two per night. He didn't sleep at all before
his Opening Day start against the San Diego Padres—even though he
had taken a sleeping pill prescribed by the Mets' trainer. Harnisch also
lost 35 pounds over the course of his depression. Some athletes in the
decades since have eloquently put forth reasons both internal and external for their struggles. But for opening up while still adjusting to taking
psychiatric medication for presumably the first time, Harnisch did a hell
of a job.

I tried to reach Harnisch and couldn't. Like many athletes who speak openly about their mental illness or other struggles (Harnisch does not like the term "mental illness" for himself: "I see [depression] mostly like a long cold, a cold in my brain"), he didn't want to be lauded. "I'm no crusader; don't give me this bold, stepping-out stuff," Harnisch told Robert Lipsyte of the *New York Times* in late 1998. "I just think a guy should do what's right, which is letting people know you can get through [a depressive episode]. You can get your life and your personality back."

And get them back Harnisch did, it would seem. He returned to the major league mound for the Mets in August 1997. For the 1998 season, he signed with the Cincinnati Reds and revitalized his career with a 3.14 earned run average. In 1999, he carried the team to the cusp of a wild-card berth (losing the one-game playoff to . . . the Mets). He played 14 major league seasons in all and over the decades since has taken jobs around the league here and there.

* * *

Elsewhere in 1990s-Mets-related mental illness lore, left-handed pitcher Bill Pulsipher said there was just one psychologist available for the entire organization at the time he was on the team. "I was also young and wild and wasn't really [receptive] as much as I probably could've or should've [been]," he said.

A second-round draft pick of New York in 1991, Pulsipher became part of Generation K: As with the other members of the much-hyped trio, Jason Isringhausen and Paul Wilson, the stakes were high for Pulsipher's call-up to the majors. He played in 1995 before sitting out to recuperate from Tommy John surgery—a procedure common for pitchers that repairs the ulnar collateral ligament—to fix his blown-out elbow. When he came back, doing rehab work in the minors, he wasn't the same. He was anxious. "My fingers didn't feel connected to my arms, and my arms didn't feel connected to my body," he reflected in 2005, his first time opening up about his mental illness. "It was absolutely surreal. My body was changing, right there on the mound, and my world would never be the same."

It wasn't just that one game, Pulsipher found. "Every five days, what once was so easy—throwing baseballs hard and accurate—became something I could no longer do. Soon I couldn't even imagine doing it," he wrote. Pulsipher, as he later told me, had butterflies. Sweaty palms. Sweaty underarms.

The anxiety was new to him and clearly centered on baseball: His symptoms would worsen as his starts neared. Of being at the stadium, he said, "The most comfortable place on the planet for you becomes the most uncomfortable place on the planet." Along with the anxiety came depression. Pulsipher would lay in bed all day until he had to get up to go to the field. "I'm hopefully dreaming about something better than what I'm thinking about when I'm awake," he said.

The Mets didn't quite know what to do with Pulsipher when he experienced these symptoms in 1998—not long after Harnisch's admission—so they sent him back to the minors for a rehab journey, first with Triple-A Norfolk. Sending someone down to the minors is (hopefully) a fix for their injury or decline in ability. But Pulsipher told the team that rather than pitching, he needed to be sorting himself out. Instead, the Mets essentially demoted him again, dumping him in extended spring training. That only made Pulsipher feel worse: Here he was, a bona fide major leaguer, struggling against much younger, unproven guys. Eventually, he asked the team doctor for help, but he took his medication for anxiety and depression only irregularly, against the doctor's orders. The Mets traded him to the Milwaukee Brewers in July 1998, kicking off many years of yo-yoing throughout the majors, minors, and other leagues.

I called up Pulsipher to interview him, yes, but also just to see how he's doing now. He played in the majors for six seasons, beginning in 1995, and in the minors and indie ball to make it a playing career totaling 20 years. I wonder all the time about athletes like him, who make headlines not for their athletic prowess but for their mental illness. "I'm living. I work. I'm not always happy about it, but I mean, who is?" he reported. The perceived failure of Generation K is still mocked to this day. (The other members didn't meet the lofty expectations set for them, either.) Pulsipher makes media appearances from time to time, but I wanted to know more.

He is living in Long Island, New York, and working in construction. Before I began recording, I explained that I was reporting and writing about mental health in sports. "That's all the rage these days, eh?" I answered in the affirmative. He clarified that he didn't mean his comment in a negative way. "I don't want to say that society is becoming weak," he said. "I think it's just people are becoming more in tune with themselves and what's going on with themselves and trying to understand what's going on, especially when you go through a period of time when you're on top of the world, you're successful, you're doing the things you know you can do, that all of a sudden you can't do, and all of a sudden you're trying to understand. And not because of a physical thing, because of a mental thing."

Pulsipher no longer takes medication for anxiety or depression. He said he still experiences both from time to time but nothing near the degree he did while pitching. If anything, his anxiety now is most prominent when he watches his kids play baseball.

It was a lonely world for Pulsipher, even as he and others like Harnisch slowly began to draw attention to baseball's mental illness problem. At the time, Pulsipher could tell something was up with the younger Rick Ankiel. The pair knew each other because Ankiel was living in Port St. Lucie, Florida, where the Mets trained. But the two, as far as Pulsipher remembers, never acknowledged their shared struggles. (Ankiel, in 2017, would write with Tim Brown *The Phenomenon: Pressure, the Yips, and the Pitch That Changed My Life*, about his own experience with anxiety as a pitcher and outfielder in the majors.) A year after Pulsipher's own disclosure, MLB Cy Young winner Zack Greinke's (social anxiety and depression) would come. In an ideal world, Pulsipher said, athletes won't have to talk publicly about mental illness the way he and others did if they don't want to. The issues can just be simply handled quietly and routinely.

But most ballplayers were reluctant to discuss their struggles and stints on medication. Pulsipher wrote in 2005 that "it's stupid, pseudo-macho garbage. Ballplayers are people, flesh and blood. We're not robots. Some might have money in their pockets, but that doesn't change the chemicals in their brains, the serotonin and norepinephrine that affect their thoughts and moods. Ballplayers aren't supposed to feel anxiety? Have you ever pitched to Barry Bonds?"

* * *

Much to Royce White's chagrin, everyone knew him as the guy who refused to get on a plane. In 2018, White rejected that characterization to me. That's when I interviewed him for a *Ringer* article about the state of mental health care in the NBA, soon after All-Stars Kevin Love and DeMar DeRozan had spoken out about their experiences with anxiety and depression, respectively. Our conversation took place six years after White was selected sixteenth in the NBA draft by the Houston Rockets. After getting suspended from and then leaving the University of Minnesota's team, he had shown a lot of promise out of Iowa State and signed a two-year, $3 million rookie contract. But White would never take the court with the Rockets during the regular season.

"Everyone involved agrees the reason for White's rapid fall from the highest levels of basketball had nothing to do with his talent, which is by all accounts NBA-worthy," wrote Mary Pilon in an expertly done 2017 *Esquire* story on the superstar who never was. She explored in depth White's disagreements with the league over how it handles—or, in his view, doesn't handle—mental health care and accommodations for athletes. There were, of course, planes involved. White had been diagnosed with OCD and generalized anxiety disorder as a teenager, and he had asked the Rockets whether he could take a bus to away games rather than a plane with the team.

"Being 30,000 feet in the air feels like you have no control," White told Pilon. "And you really don't. In a bus, I can gauge speed. I can gauge environment because I can see out of the windows, I can see what's going on. In the plane, you got this little window that you can see out of left, or you may be able to get across the row and see out of the plane right, but you don't know what else is out there."

The NBA reportedly told the Rockets, who, White said, were initially accommodating, that providing alternative transportation for him might violate the league's salary cap. White did not attend Houston's games that fall, and then he initially refused a reassignment to what was then called the D-League (now the G League), a feeder system for the NBA like MLB's minor leagues.

He said in 2013 that he hadn't asked for a bus to *every* away game, just when possible. "The media shaped it like I'm this anxious kid and I need all this special help, but it wasn't about that," White said. "It was about creating a policy for people who have mental health disorders." The NBA, at the time, didn't have one. White ultimately played in 16 D-League games that season for the Rio Grande Valley Vipers. The only playing time he saw in the NBA was three games for the Sacramento Kings in 2014. He scored zero points.

L. Jon Wertheim, writing for *Sports Illustrated* in 2020 as White took up a short-lived MMA career, reported that the athlete felt he was blackballed from the NBA due to his friction with the league over mental health accommodations. But his impact was felt deeply in his first professional sport. As one former NBA general manager told Wertheim, "I'm still not sure how good he was as a basketball player. But if we're talking moving the needle in terms of getting comfortable talking about anxiety and mental health, he's a Curt Flood–type figure." (Flood was a professional baseball player and activist best known as the father of MLB free agency.)

Before taking up MMA, White played basketball in Canada and Europe. Reflecting back on his brief NBA career, he told Wertheim, "You know, I had everything to gain by not even saying anything about mental health. Actually, I was advised by my agent and by other people in the basketball world to not go public and talk about mental health at all. Because I was in line to make a couple hundred million dollars. But I said, 'Hey, mental health is a conversation we need to [have].' And I am living proof that people with anxiety not only aren't weak, but they can be profoundly strong."

In recent years, White has taken a heel turn, depending on your politics. A 2022 *Mother Jones* feature asked, "What Happened to Royce White?" It's a question I'd been asking myself that year, too. In February 2022, White had announced that he was running for the House of Representatives as a Republican in Minnesota, hoping to vie for Democrat Ilhan Omar's seat.

At the start of a two-minute, 20-second video attached to White's announcement tweet, a 2013 *New York Times* headline flickered across the screen: "A Player with a Cause, but without a Team." Then after some praise from pundits came White's own narration. "Ten years ago, I took on the NBA and the establishment," he said. "I said that mental health was one of the greatest issues we face, and I was willing to give up my dream to fight for people I had never met."

Even as his political ideology seems to have moved drastically to the right of where it was even a couple of years before, when he was speaking out about George Floyd's murder by a Minneapolis police officer, he was calling on people to remember his past in a positive light, to think of him as a leader. (Although it was maybe less of a pivot than it seemed, as White said in 2022: "What I was protesting [after Floyd's death] was that we were living under the thumb of a corporatocracy . . . this sort of merger of government and corporations at the world scale. The NBA is the perfect representation of that.") He was also calling on people to see him as someone who had fought for the greater good. In a way, he had. But that did start with relaying his own anxieties and making his stance personal.

Regardless of his changing views, it's clear that White is still proud of the stand he took against the NBA a decade before his primary election. He elaborated on his announcement to run for office in a winding, bigotry-filled, 3,500-word Substack newsletter. "I spoke up about mental health and anxiety because it's the greatest social issue of our time," White wrote in between many, many jabs at Democrats and various aspects of their "woke politics." He's right about that. He spoke up for not only anyone who may have been struggling with mental illness back then, but also athletes who are struggling now.

In 2018, the Cleveland Cavaliers' Kevin Love tweeted his thanks at White, who two years later repaid the gesture by criticizing Love, speaking to *Time*: "The difference was I challenged the status quo," White said. "I challenged policy. He didn't challenge policy. And it's not by accident that the American media would prop up a figure who wouldn't challenge the fundamental structure of society." (Love experienced a panic attack during a basketball game in 2017 and wrote about it the next year in *The*

Players' Tribune, helping to kick-start a wave of renewed discussion about mental illness in the NBA and more broadly across sports. Love has since collaborated with the league on mental health public service announcements, though he also freely acknowledges there's more work to be done.)

Mother Jones described White's politics, as of the summer of 2022, as "tinfoil hat populism." Writer Eamon Whalen explained, "He believes that the Democrats, Bill Gates, the World Economic Forum, President Xi Jinping, the CCP, non-MAGA Republicans, George Soros, 'millennial purple-haired white liberal women,' 'the Church of LGBTQ,' the National Basketball Association, and various government agencies all act on behalf of the same 'global corporate community.'" His mentor, it may not surprise you to know after reading the above, is none other than former Donald Trump administration chief strategist Steve Bannon. The two met in part through a connection White made while playing Big3 basketball (a three-on-three league founded by Ice Cube and his business partner). White would go on to appear on Bannon's programs at least 25 times by the spring of 2022.

Later that year, White lost his primary campaign by 11 percentage points, not even getting the chance to directly battle Omar for her seat in the November general election. I tried my best to talk to White. I wanted to hear for myself how and why his politics has changed, how he looks back on his disagreement with the NBA, and how he sees his legacy at this moment. My attempts to reach him directly went unanswered. Through his campaign in the spring before his primary, we set up an interview, but he never called at the scheduled time. My efforts to reschedule were met with radio silence.

White is a good reminder that not all pioneers share the same goals or politics. But in 2018, when we spoke for *The Ringer*, he passed on an NFL metaphor regarding our current mental health dialogue in sports that I think is worth considering no matter your views: "We are first-and-40, and we're acting like a 10-yard pass is anything other than us still being 30 yards behind where we need to be," White said. "It needs to be acknowledged that we are re-having a conversation that we already had."

* * *

Michael Phelps is the most storied athlete of these mental health pioneers in sports. He's also a relative latecomer compared with the others in this chapter, having first gone in depth on his substance abuse in 2015 in a *Sports Illustrated* interview with Tim Layden.

As Phelps was racking up hardware—28 Olympic medals in all—he was sinking even deeper into his dark thoughts. After the 2012 Games in London, he later told David Axelrod in a forum, he "didn't want to be in the sport anymore. . . . I didn't want to be alive anymore." Publicly, at least, his situation kept worsening. In September 2014, he drove erratically at 84 miles per hour in a 45-mile-per-hour zone in Baltimore. His blood alcohol level was clocked at 0.14, well above the 0.08 legal limit. He pleaded guilty to a drunk-driving charge that December. That guilty plea came a decade after another one, that time for driving while impaired, and five years after a British tabloid published a photo of him smoking a bong.

"I was in a really dark place," Phelps told Layden about the 2014 arrest and the journalists camping outside his house afterward. Shortly after that arrest, with the support of friends and family, Phelps checked himself into The Meadows, a residential rehabilitation treatment center in the Arizona desert. (He wasn't the first athlete to venture to the Wickenburg facility; Los Angeles Dodgers pitcher Bob Welch, for one, had been to the same facility decades earlier for alcohol use.) The swimmer had no cell phone or internet access, though he was allowed to make calls each night.

"I wound up uncovering a lot of things about myself that I probably knew, but I didn't want to approach," he told Layden about his time there. "One of them was that for a long time, I saw myself as the athlete that I was, but not as a human being. I would be in sessions with complete strangers who know exactly who I am, but they don't respect me for things I've done, but instead for who I am as a human being. I found myself feeling happier and happier."

Reflecting on that 2015 *Sports Illustrated* cover story to me in 2022 for the same publication, Phelps doesn't even know what drew him to share so much in that initial chat. "I don't even know the question that Tim asked that made me just feel comfortable and safe and confident in opening up," he said. Phelps thinks it's one of the "rawest" interviews he's ever given.

He only grew more and more outspoken after his 2016 retirement. Two years later, Phelps reflected at length on his career and his feelings throughout it during that 20-minute conversation with Axelrod in front of a hushed Chicago crowd at the Kennedy Forum conference, which was focused on behavioral health. "You do contemplate suicide," he said, by then no stranger to talking about athletes' deaths and his own past thoughts about it. That is a good thing, experts say, and it potentially gets the conversation going for people who might be experiencing suicidal thoughts themselves. And the talk helps him, too: "For me, the more I share my stories, the lower my shoulders drop, the more comfortable I am about my story and about who I am," Phelps told me in 2022.

"Really, after every Olympics I think I fell into a major state of depression," Phelps said to Axelrod back in 2018. That cycle began in 2004, Phelps explained, in the fall following the Athens Games. (Phelps's Olympic career had started four years earlier, in Sydney, when the 15-year-old came home without a medal after notching an impressive fifth place in the 200-meter butterfly.)

Phelps took his outspokenness on elite athlete mental health to a new level in 2020, when HBO Sports released *The Weight of Gold*, a documentary about Olympians' struggles narrated by the legendary swimmer. "I can't see any more suicides," he told the *New York Times* in promoting the film's debut. That line, like the film as a whole, can be seen as a direct challenge to the USOPC to take better care of its athletes' minds.

Movingly, alongside many athletes still among us, the documentary features posthumous appearances from decorated U.S. bobsledder Steven Holcomb, who died, possibly by suicide, in 2017 at age 37. It's not until near the end of the film that Holcomb's death is revealed. "Holcomb was the best bobsled pilot of his generation," wrote Andy Bull for *The Guardian*. "He measured his success by inches and regretted every little error." Holcomb spoke in the film about surviving depression and a 2007 suicide attempt.

Phelps drove his point home hard as *The Weight of Gold*'s narrator: "What else has to happen for this to change? . . . Do five other athletes have to [die by suicide] to see change? How far down the road are we going to get before somebody stands up and says, 'We have to do something.'" It's rhetoric he uses often (see the *Times* interview he did above), but it always reads as genuine to me. Deep down, you get the sense, he knows that a story like Holcomb's could've been his.

Seven years after Phelps started disclosing bits and pieces of his history with mental illness, did he feel rehabilitated, as that *Sports Illustrated* cover suggested? I asked him. "It's probably an ongoing process," Phelps said. "I don't know if I will ever understand myself completely, but I will continue to try. I think that process has allowed me to become who I am today. I'm very thankful for it. I would say we're on a better journey than I think we were seven years ago—definitely mentally. I know what the word *communication* is and I know how to do it, whereas seven years ago I'm not really sure I could've spelled it."

* * *

These pioneers, from Harnisch and Pulsipher to Holdsclaw and White to Phelps and way beyond, span decades and genders and sports. But they were all left without enough tools to handle their mental illness. (And who among us, even with a new, high-end set of tools, can quickly and adeptly fix a complex problem stemming from inside ourselves *and* from systemic failures?) They were thrust onto big stages and summoned the confidence within themselves to speak out, either during their playing years or shortly after, no matter the potential consequences in their industry or the public eye. And they all survived—sometimes even thrived—in spite of the odds stacked against them.

Each time one of these pioneers said something, they paved the way for future generations of athletes, both stars and supporting players, to build on those disclosures and help the nonathletes among us find the strength within ourselves to ask for help and show vulnerability. They don't owe us that, by the way. As Schuck wrote about Harnisch, not all of those statements were perfect representations of what could be said that get at the crux of inner turmoil and systemic injustice. And the statements that come next never will be, either. Don't forget the roots, as imperfect as they may be, as we look forward to where the mental health movement (if we can even call it one cohesive movement) in sports has carried us. Wave after wave of athletes would join a cause they'd probably rather have sat out.

CHAPTER 5

Open the Floodgates

More Athletes Join the Cause

THE NEXT PHASE OF THE REVOLUTION WE'RE CHRONICLING IN ATHLETE mental health care arguably tipped off with two men, both NBA players. Following the pioneers—like Michael Phelps and Chamique Holdsclaw—by years or even sometimes decades, this new wave of heartfelt stories is distinct because it reenergized the somewhat dormant conversation around mental health in sports. It was a dialogue, it seemed, that fans were willing to consider more deeply when two beloved basketball stars weighed in through social media and athlete-driven media, respectively. Mental health disclosures throughout sports, as we'll see, are easier and maybe even more compelling to fans in the digital era.

A tweet appeared—as many stories start these days—in late winter 2018. "This depression get the best of me," DeMar DeRozan posted early in the morning on February 17, during All-Star weekend.[1] You can imagine him up late, as most of the United States and Canada slept, wondering what fans and others might think in the morning as they scrolled through their feeds from bed and read his vulnerable admission. But DeRozan didn't really think there would be much of a response at all, he later told me. He was typing a lyric from rapper Kevin Gates's song "Tomorrow," yes, but it also turned out to represent how the All-Star forward—then with the Toronto Raptors—said he felt at the time he tweeted it.

"It's one of them things that no matter how indestructible we look like we are, we're all human at the end of the day," DeRozan, then 28, told Doug Smith of the *Toronto Star* about a week after his tweet. "We all got feelings . . . all of that. Sometimes . . . it gets the best of you, where times everything in the whole world's on top of you." He continued, acknowledging his own reluctance to talk about the depression he'd experienced since he was a kid, but also about the importance of getting over that hump. "It's not nothing I'm against or ashamed of," DeRozan said. "Now, at my age, I understand how many people go through it. Even if it's just somebody can look at it like, 'He goes through it and he's still out there being successful and doing this,' I'm okay with that."[2]

There was a lifetime of struggle behind DeRozan's message. "I think I had just hit my wall emotionally with everything that was going on with me just in life, from being a teenager to being an adult, just everything catching up to me," he told me in 2023. "I didn't think nothing of it till I woke up the next day and see how much of a conversation it started." DeRozan wasn't tweeting with the goal of reigniting any sort of dialogue around mental illness in sports—he just wanted to get some feelings off his chest.

What Smith wrote of DeRozan after he stepped forward was sharp: "That [the tweet] came out of nowhere in the dark of the night, on an NBA all-star weekend many thought would be a celebration for the Compton kid at home, was jarring. It was out of character and out of place, but not as it happens out of the norm. It set off a maelstrom of support throughout social media, and tossing it off just as a lyric from a song is to not do the whole issue justice."[3]

To boil down someone's deepest, most personal thoughts into a single tweet would not fully capture the situation with that person alone and certainly not with the mental health crisis throughout the NBA, elite sports leagues, or society at large. The tweet, thanks to Smith's interview and what was to come from a peer of DeRozan's, would not live in a vacuum. "He changed a billion-dollar business" is the simple yet grand way Raptors guard Fred VanVleet, a former teammate of DeRozan's, contextualized the tweet to journalists in 2020. "He changed it pretty much single-handedly [by] speaking out."[4]

* * *

On March 6, 2018, Cleveland Cavaliers power forward and center Kevin Love—also an All-Star—wrote an essay for *The Players' Tribune*, the Derek Jeter–founded, athlete-driven online publication, about his own experiences with mental illness. It was called "Everyone Is Going through Something." Love cut right to the chase. In the middle of a home game the previous fall versus the Atlanta Hawks, he had experienced a panic attack. It was his first, so he didn't understand what was happening. All he knew is that he felt winded near the start of the game, which was unusual. By the time a third-quarter time-out came around, his heart was racing. "Everything was spinning, like my brain was trying to climb out of my head," he wrote.[5] Instead of getting back into the game and pushing through his discomfort, Love ran to the locker room and ended up lying on the floor of the training room, trying to breathe.

Love didn't know what was wrong with him on that fall day. His medical tests at the Cleveland Clinic checked out. But then where did that leave him? All he knew is that he had wanted to keep what had happened to himself, save for the few members of the organization who already knew. "Call it a stigma or call it fear or insecurity—you can call it a number of things—but what I was worried about wasn't just my own inner struggles but how difficult it was to *talk about* them," Love wrote in that *Players' Tribune* piece. "I didn't want people to perceive me as somehow less reliable as a teammate, and it all went back to the playbook I'd learned growing up."[6]

The Cavs quietly helped Love find a therapist, and over time, he started to break down the shame he felt was preventing him from speaking up. Eventually, Love's panic attack and subsequent experiences changed the way he saw everything about mental health and himself. "For 29 years, I thought about mental health as someone else's problem," he wrote. "Sure, I knew on some level that some people benefited from asking for help or opening up. I just never thought it was for me. To me, it was [a] form of weakness that could derail my success in sports or make me seem weird or different."[7]

Finally coming forward, Love told me in the fall of 2022—more than four years after the fact—"was what I needed so much at the time. It was something that helped save me and the idea of who I really am in my skin. That just allowed me to stop living in the shadows."

Love went on in the 2018 essay to detail his early journey with his therapist—he was still seeing one at the time we spoke—which he called "terrifying and awkward and hard."[8] Importantly, he also cited DeRozan's disclosure as a reason he felt comfortable coming forward with his own. (DeRozan shared the sentiment right back the day after Love's essay was published: "Much respect to @kevinlove!!!!" DeRozan tweeted.)[9] Together, the two of them helped usher in a new wave of athletes speaking up about their mental illness.

Asked years later why he thinks his and Love's words touched so many people, DeRozan said, "We don't realize we hide behind so much stuff emotionally that we neglect our own feelings at times, and for me I think it just resonated because that's just how everybody feels. A lot of people wouldn't say it, especially people that get held at a certain pedestal or feel like they have it all or have a bunch of money—[we're] just showing that that isn't the answer, either. We all go through things, and just to show how human we are in the same token spoke volumes."

So we know that the conversation around mental health and mental illness in sports had never been more robust and wide ranging than it was toward the latter half of the 2010s, thanks to DeRozan, Love, and scores of others. But why? Why were fans and reporters and teammates and families and friends better prepared to listen now than they may have been before? What made athletes feel more comfortable coming forward? And how did they spread their messages more effectively?

* * *

When Love and I spoke, he was eager to funnel a lot of the credit for speaking up and the progress that ensued DeRozan's way, recognizing that the former Toronto star's disclosure was perhaps even tougher to make than his own. "He has that quiet confidence demeanor about him. At the time, he was a mid-to-late 20s Black man in America from

Compton, California," said Love, who is white. "For him to come out and say that he struggles with depression, there's even maybe more of a stigma behind that." (DeRozan doesn't exactly agree with that assessment: "[Mental illness is] something that hurts. It drags you down. It puts you in a dark place, no matter who you are. The feeling of depression does not discriminate versus anybody.")

Love also recognizes that his own spot in the national and even international discourse around mental illness in sports is significant and places him among some other greats. "I'm just very thankful and grateful for [DeRozan] but also the outpouring of love that we both shared in after the fact. There are so many people before, like Michael Phelps and a number of others, and so many people after the fact, like the Simone Bileses, the Dak Prescotts, the Naomi Osakas, so many people in the public eye."

The reaction to the disclosures from Love and DeRozan was swift and overwhelmingly positive. "The last week has been one of the most incredible things that I have witnessed, period," DeRozan said shortly after his disclosure. "Everything I got back from it was so positive."[10] He also called himself a "sacrificial lamb"—in a good way, clarifying that it was worth it if he could help other people, like Love, share their stories.[11] (It was also worth it for DeRozan's own health. "You have a clearer mind, and you have a different type of stance of knowing yourself," he told the *Washington Post* in the spring of 2022 as he led the Chicago Bulls into their first postseason since 2017. "Not feeling like you're behind the curtain, it gives you a sense of freedom."[12])

In 2018, the stories and support for DeRozan and Love kept flooding in. Within the NBA, Kelly Oubre Jr., then playing for the Washington Wizards, echoed his colleagues' sentiments and said he could relate to their experiences with depression and anxiety. "We're normal human beings," Oubre said on a local NBC podcast. "We face a lot more adversity, a lot more problems. . . . It's a little bit more amped up, we just can't show it. I feel like people who are on the outside looking in don't really understand because they see us as superheroes, but we're normal people, man. We go through the issues that normal people go through times 10."[13]

Golden State Warriors coach Steve Kerr offered in response to Love's disclosure, "We're all human beings. We all have our own story, we all have our own lives, and nobody's is perfect. So, everybody's got things and you need friends and you need support and you need help to get through everything."[14] Even LeBron James shouted out Love, his then teammate on the Cavaliers, on Twitter the day his essay was published, writing (alongside some upbeat emoji), "You're even more powerful now than ever before @kevinlove!!! Salute and respect brother!"[15]

DeRozan, who said his depression "comes and goes," told me he was glad to have the support of his teammates and those around the league. Since 2018, he said, his relationship with Love has deepened. "Every time we see each other, we just embrace each other for the strength we both have to be able to share our story," DeRozan said. "I've definitely had more in-depth conversations with a lot of guys on how to get through certain things in life. That's definitely a cool thing to be able to have that type of dialogue with people, open up, and you can ask them questions and be able to help with whatever it is that they're going through."

Outside the NBA, figures across sports were taking notice, too. The WNBA's Layshia Clarendon was quick to cite Love when I asked them who they remember looking up to for inspiration around mental health disclosures in sports. Taylor Ricci, a former Oregon State gymnast who cofounded Dam Worth It, a campaign to reduce stigma among athletes on her campus, recalled to me that Love's connection to the Portland area set an inspiring example for her and her peers. "He became a huge role model for us."

Not only were others across sports taking in what DeRozan and Love were saying, they were also speaking up about their own experiences. In the NHL, then–New York Islanders goaltender Robin Lehner talked candidly in 2018 about his bipolar I disorder, PTSD, and history of substance use. Writing for *The Athletic*, he explained, "For a long time, I always lived at the extremes mentally—manic and hyper-manic and depressed."[16] He wanted to die, he wrote, and he hid parts of what he was going through from everyone, even his wife. He felt much better after rehab, though, and after getting support from people inside hockey and out.

Meanwhile, in the WNBA, then–Dallas Wings star Skylar Diggins-Smith spoke in 2019 about the postpartum depression she had experienced the year before, calling out the league and the broader community for what she saw as a lack of support. "People called me a quitter, said I gave up on my team, etc., etc.," Diggins-Smith tweeted (her account has since been deleted). "Not knowing I took two FULL months away from everything because of postpartum depression. With limited resources to help me be successful mentally/physically."[17]

In 2018, ESPN had surveyed 37 female athletes across nine sports: 32 percent said they had experienced postpartum depression. Also in 2018, tennis legend Serena Williams disclosed what she calls "postpartum emotions."[18] She's talked openly over the years about other periods of mental health struggles, too.

Even in the NFL, a league often thought of as more conservative than its peers, change was on the way. There might not be a robust, league-wide movement yet, but in 2019, Indianapolis Colts co-owner and vice chair Kalen Jackson was tasked with brainstorming a new initiative for the franchise to get behind. Due to her own lifelong history of anxiety and her father's (co-owner Jim Irsay's) with substance use disorder, she and her family conceived of Kicking the Stigma—a mental health awareness campaign that would also offer grants to Indiana and national groups that raise awareness or provide treatment services. Just over two years later, in October 2022, they had given over $4.1 million to 38 recipients. They'd also raised over $17 million.

Importantly, Jackson and the Colts didn't just preach awareness and acceptance outwardly. They looked inward at their own organization as well to see how they could help not just athletes, but also coaches and front-office staff. (The Colts have had a licensed mental health professional on staff since 2015.) "As we launched this, we had to look inside at ourselves and say, *Are we providing enough?*" Jackson told me in the fall of 2022. "And we weren't." Among other things, they didn't have an employee assistance program to help workers with substance use and mental health–related issues. They've since put one in place.

One day, Jackson would love to see mental health awareness become an NFL-wide initiative because she recognizes the legitimacy that comes with the league's stamp of approval. But for now, the change her team is creating is enough for her. Star linebacker Shaquille Leonard started speaking out about his experience with grief and stress in college and afterward. Jackson also said people in Indianapolis have called the front office since Kicking the Stigma was put in place, asking for mental health advice, such as which hospital they should take a struggling family member to. Jackson clarified that despite being several years into the campaign, the Colts are still not the experts—but they are well connected with some across the state. In a league where more and more players like Leonard have been coming forward about their own experiences, offering that support—both financially and not—is a start.

* * *

Mike Delayo, a Penn State graduate student researching the rhetoric of popular culture through sport, wrote in his 2021 master's thesis, "Athletes are using digital media to construct and present their identities and amplify their voices on their own terms in ways that previous generations simply could not."[19] He has a name for this in professional athletics: "digital mental health disclosures."

"As long as the stories are being told, I think there's a value in it," Delayo said. He stressed that that's true whether athletes are talking to the media, posting on their own social accounts, or going to non-journalistic first-person sites like *The Players' Tribune*. That publication's editor in chief, Sean Patrick Conboy, talked to me in the fall of 2022 about how Love's essay and many others on the platform have helped the conversation about mental health in sports explode.

"If you would've told me eight years ago when we started the whole project that we would have John Wall just the other day speaking in very vivid detail about nearly taking his own life, it would've just seemed absolutely impossible at that time," he said. "It would've seemed almost foolish to see that as part of our strategy because we were so far away from it in the culture, just the way that all of that stuff was spoken about or, really, just not even spoken about. I would say the biggest thing in 2014, when we were launching, is that mental health was just, it wasn't even that it was stigmatized, it was just that there was no conversation going on. The very few things that would come out, it was mostly smaller athletes or athletes in sports outside of the big five. It almost would kind of be with a whimper."

Conboy pointed to Larry Sanders's 2015 video and words for the publication as what really got things going for *The Players' Tribune* on the mental health front. The Milwaukee Bucks center had stepped away from the team the year before, leading to all kinds of speculation about what he was up to. He was struggling with anxiety and getting treatment for it at a hospital program centered on mood disorders. "It taught me a lot about myself," he said. "It taught me a lot about what's important and where I want to devote my time and energy." Sanders stressed in the video that he loved basketball but felt it was "consuming too much of my life and time."[20] Conboy felt Sanders's openness ignited something in others across sports. "Pretty quickly after that, we just started getting a lot of athletes reaching out to us or their people reaching out to us saying they were dealing with something and they wanted to talk about it," Conboy said.

The art of the *Players' Tribune* disclosure is interesting. While there's no one playbook, since Conboy and his team like athletes to lead the way in telling their own stories, he stressed that they aren't going for fairy-tale endings. "We want these to be not closed books," Conboy said. "No, we're not trying to tell people that mental health is this thing where you go through something and then you get all better and you're perfect. As we all know, that's not how it is." To wit, speaking to Mirin Fader at *The Ringer* in 2022, about four years after his tweet, DeRozan would acknowledge that depression isn't something to fully get over and move past. "It don't work like that," he said. "You never just completely beat something and be totally fine."[21] That's a key point that we have seen with others, too, including Phelps and Holdsclaw.

Today, the list of current and former athletes who have used *The Players' Tribune* as a vehicle for sharing their mental health journeys with sports fans everywhere is quite long. It includes basketball players like Wall and Kayla McBride, NHL players like Daniel Carcillo, the NFL's

Brandon Marshall, and so many others. The website even has a landing page for all its stories on the topic.

Love's 2018 essay in particular resonated with people, Conboy argued, because of its specificity in describing his panic attack and subsequent emotions: "How many of us, even if you go back, you're like, *Yeah, you know, five years ago when I was at that restaurant and I thought I had heartburn or whatever. Was I having a panic attack? I was kind of stressed at the time.* And you start to be like *huh*, because some of this stuff isn't so obvious, especially when you're talking about anxiety."

When Conboy shared his restaurant example, I immediately recalled one of my own. I had been traveling in Florida with my father a few weeks after Love's essay went live. I was hypomanic at the time, largely unable to sleep and constantly recalling unpleasant childhood memories. As I began to eat dinner out, my throat tightened up. I couldn't breathe. My dad and I left the restaurant and went to a nearby hospital, where I was shut in a small room without a bed and not given an IV—a clear sign the professionals thought this was all in my head. I felt ignored. Nothing was wrong with me, I was told. It was only in hindsight, as I finished work (yes, I went straight back to work after that incident) on a *Ringer* story about the state of mental health care in the NBA in light of DeRozan's and Love's disclosures, that it occurred to me I had likely suffered a panic attack.

The next year, yet another *Players' Tribune* piece made a splash. In August 2019, then-WNBA and Australia star Liz Cambage joined the contributors' list. Her piece "DNP-Mental Health"[22] (read: "did not play") is widely regarded as a key essay in the awareness movement and push for change in health care for athletes. She wrote about the depression and anxiety that she, then almost 28, had "battled for about half my life." Cambage also wrote of spending nearly every night of her rookie season, with the Tulsa Shock in 2011, in tears and of being put on suicide watch in 2016. The title of her essay is a reference to what she feels as though her injury report should've read for a couple of games she missed while playing for the Las Vegas Aces shortly before the piece was published; instead, it read "DNP-Rest."

"I know that, on the surface, people are 'ready' to talk about mental health. But are they *really*?" she wrote,[23] directly challenging her readers. As Delayo recounted in his thesis two years later, "She almost taunts the audience . . . resembling a coach trying to motivate her team to take their game a step further."[24]

Cambage is not a gold-star example (not that there is such a thing) of a role-model athlete making a mental health disclosure and inspiring the masses. She's continued to speak out about her struggles but simultaneously has also seemingly tarnished her own reputation by calling Nigerian basketball players "monkeys," telling them to "go back to their third-world countries," and slapping one of them across the face in 2021, ahead of the Tokyo Olympics, according to a *Sunday Telegraph* investigation that featured accounts from anonymous Nigerian players. (Cambage has denied the reports.)

At the time, before the news came out, Cambage cited mental health reasons for stepping down from her spot on the Australian national team. Mental illness, it should not need to be said, is not an excuse for colorism, assault, verbal abuse, or any other bad behavior. But the points she raised in her essay, the challenge to dig deep and go beyond awareness when thinking about the future of mental health care for athletes, are still valid. "While both Kevin Love and DeMar DeRozan famously told their stories about navigating mental illness (anxiety and depression, respectively), which opened the NBA's own boundaries around discussing mental health, this was the first time that a WNBA player had gone out on a limb so publicly and didn't hold back," Jackie Powell wrote for *Sports Illustrated* in 2021.[25]

It was a "wakeup call," Terri Jackson, the executive director of the league's players association, told Powell.[26] It's not that female athletes are necessarily discouraged by society from making the kinds of statements that DeRozan and Love had, but I do think it's harder for them to do so and receive a so-called hero's welcome. That's partly because there's far less media coverage of women's sports than men's, which are more established due to systemic sexism, and perhaps also partly because women are more commonly *expected* to have complex emotional reactions compared with their male peers. When women show what people believe to be signs of weakness, they're not surprised. It doesn't necessarily rock their worldviews the same way masculine athletes like DeRozan and Love expressing "weakness" might.

Of *The Players' Tribune* and other public statements from athletes about their mental health, Delayo told me, "I'm optimistic that the next generations of athletes growing up will be able to say, oh yeah, this athlete whose poster I have on my wall—assuming that posters remain a thing for the next generation—talked about the performance anxiety they had throughout their career. Maybe someone like me is able to channel, *Hey, if you're feeling this way, that's okay.*"

* * *

Former NHL and Team Canada goalie Corey Hirsch also used *The Players' Tribune* to tell his story. In 2017, he opened up about his OCD in an extremely well-titled essay ("Dark, Dark, Dark, Dark, Dark, Dark, Dark, Dark"). He was diagnosed with the mental illness during his time in the NHL, about 20 years before his essay, but didn't come forward due to the stigma and a fear of losing his job. In the summer of 1994, he wanted to die. He planned to drive his sports car as fast as it would go off a cliff. He hit 140 miles per hour before skidding to a halt, solely because he was afraid of what would happen if he followed through but *didn't* die and had to deal with severe injuries. "That image was so terrifying that, somehow, it seemed worse than death."[27] So he vowed to get help, eventually confiding in a trainer about the dark thoughts he'd obsessed over.

He described OCD to me thusly: "It's 24 hours a day, seven days a week. It's relentless. And along with every thought comes a taser gun of anxiety, almost like a tsunami wave of anxiety, and anxiety fills the thought, so it's just one big circle. It's like you're fighting with yourself, and your own brain just keeps torturing you."

When it came to telling the personal details of his story, Hirsch, who in 2021 began cohosting a podcast about mental health in sports called *Blindsided* with *The Players' Tribune*, selected his initial avenue of public disclosure carefully. "What I know through my own dealings with *The Players' Tribune* is how kind, how empathetic, how compassionate they are about telling people's stories," he said. "And there's never a 'got you' moment in a *Players' Tribune*–type article. It's always: How can we use this to help somebody else?"

As Hirsch suggests, *The Players' Tribune* itself sits in a somewhat odd, liminal space between straight journalism and straight-from-the-athletes'-mouth (or keyboard) disclosures on, say, Instagram or Twitter. (Conboy called it a "complement to media.") For Delayo, those blurred lines are part of what makes the website so compelling. And all three methods above—straight journalism write-ups like long-form profiles, *The Players' Tribune* and similar widely published personal essays, and social media posts—are different from the opportunities from decades past that athletes like Pete Harnisch had in traditional press conferences to share their stories. (Those events, Delayo reasoned, were "the only time in the 20th century when athletes were given a forum to talk about things, even [as] it was extremely mediated and they had a limited amount of agency.")

There's also the matter of making room for disclosures across formats and platforms. Delayo argued that in the digital age, there's an infinite amount of space for storytelling where before there were clear constraints. "Some of these disclosures that we have been able to read and sympathize with, we just wouldn't have had access to without digital media," he said. "Not because we didn't want to hear those stories but because they weren't going to be presented to us in the one to two hours of *SportsCenter* or the x amount of words that fit in a newspaper sports section."

Now, of course, *SportsCenter*, along with print and digital sports sections nationwide, does more regularly tackle mental health–related subjects. There's a definite domino effect: The more disclosures there are, the more there likely will continue to be because we're reducing stigma and signaling to readers, listeners, and viewers that these issues their idols are grappling with truly matter. When fans show their interest and investment in those stories, media outlets and athletes pay attention. They know there's an audience—an increasingly big and supportive one—for storytelling around mental illness. Cynically speaking, a lot of entities might tell those mental health stories at least in part for capitalistic reasons instead of or in addition to because it's the morally right thing to do, but the outcome, nonetheless, tends to be a good one.

* * *

When athletes tell their stories candidly and in detail, no matter the medium, they, in an ideal world, end up challenging sports teams, leagues, and governing bodies to take action. Also in an ideal world, those entities actually rise to the challenge and give athletes the care they need and deserve. While our world is far from ideal, it's true that ever since DeRozan, Love, and many of their peers opened the floodgates near the end of the 2010s, professional sports leagues have made significant strides in tending to athletes' mental health.

Leading into the 2019 season, the NFL and the NFL players association came to a joint agreement that each team would have to retain a behavioral health team physician who would be available to players at their facility for a minimum of eight to 12 hours a week. The agreement also required each team to have a mental health emergency action plan. These requirements are meant to supplement the NFL Life Line, implemented back in 2012, which players, coaches, staff, and family members can call or chat to speak with a trained counselor. For a league in which head injuries are pervasive, this step seems particularly important as the start of what needs to happen.

Chris Carr, the Green Bay Packers' full-time director of performance psychology and team behavior health clinician, joined the team before the joint agreement was put in place. When he first started studying sport psychology 30-something years ago, "there was a jungle, and [athletes] wanted a road cut in it. That's where I started, with a machete in my hand," he reflected to me in 2021. He feels supported by his team, to the point where its longtime star signal-caller, Aaron Rodgers, openly advocated for mental health awareness, Carr said. "In all the years of [my] practice, the role of sport psychology is being embraced, and the role of mental health in athletics is being embraced more than I've ever seen it."

To Carr's point, the NFL is far from the only league engaging in such initiatives. The home of DeRozan and Love, the NBA, is on a similar course. Before the 2019–2020 season, the league went a little further than the NFL in mandating that each team have at least one *full-time* psychologist or behavioral health therapist on staff. The NBA also required that each team retain a licensed psychiatrist when necessary. "It all started with having a licensed therapist on every team, but I think the next part is really helping people understand the resources that not only they have for themselves [but also] their family," Love told me.

The NBA players association has a mental health and wellness program as well. Earlier in 2019, about a year after DeRozan and Love spoke out, league commissioner Adam Silver said at the MIT Sloan Sports Analytics Conference, "When I meet with [players], what surprises me is that they're truly unhappy. A lot of these young men are generally unhappy."[28] As of the 2021 season, the NBA's sister league, the WNBA, requires each team to retain one or two licensed mental health professionals. Athletes, including players association executive council president Nneka Ogwumike, believe there's still a long way to go.

Other leagues are a bit later to the game but still putting forth an effort. The National Women's Soccer League (NWSL) and the players association finally agreed to their first collective bargaining agreement at the beginning of 2022. The historic document addresses a lot of issues that indirectly and directly affect players' mental health, like ensuring they'll earn a living wage for the first time in the league's 10-year history. On the mental health front, specifically, players are granted up to six months of paid leave. Also per the agreement, each team is required to retain the services of at least one clinician—a licensed psychiatrist or psychologist with at least five years of experience working with multicultural populations.

Such requirements are essential in a league that, in between some seasons, has had only a short break between the NWSL championship game and the next year's training camp before the Challenge Cup tournament (which was born in the pandemic and has shifted time frames). "Breaks are important, you know?" OL Reign forward and 2019 Rookie of the Year Bethany Balcer told me. "Some people take vacations. In our sport, it's hard to do that at times. . . . We've had a two-month offseason, and sometimes I feel like it's not long enough to mentally recharge."

Balcer praised Christen Press, a U.S. women's national team star and the first player signed to expansion team Angel City FC, for taking time off from the game as a mental health break. "It's important to know yourself and your limits," Balcer stressed.

I talked to another NWSL player, Gabby Kessler, in 2022. She would retire from the Houston Dash almost immediately afterward. Kessler was on medication to manage her anxiety, depression, and ADHD after having long resisted help. "I remember driving into practice being like, *What if I just drove my car into this fence right now?*" she said. "Like, that's not a normal thought to have." Other elite athletes opening up helped her to as well on social media, in journalistic interviews, and in talks with her coaches. Kessler's therapy and psychiatry appointments were in network, but she knew another player in the NWSL who had been paying upward of $100 per therapy session before the collective bargaining agreement (CBA) was ratified.

Balcer herself has experienced performance-related panic attacks while on the pitch as well as before and after games. Immediately after she started having them, in her sophomore season with the team, the club brought aboard a sport psychologist, she said—more than a year before the CBA required one. These resources are especially crucial in a league that has historically not treated its athletes well. Reports of abuse were rife within the NWSL, and it would take years and years for some of the bad actors, including many head coaches and owners, to get ousted and the allegations to be made public.

Press took that monthslong mental health break from soccer starting in the fall of 2021—*seven* years after she started raising alarms about emotionally abusive behavior she described from then–Chicago Red Stars head coach Rory Dames. "There's this general consensus in sport that you just suffer: You push through it and keep going and that's what makes you tough and that's what makes you an athlete," Press told *GQ*'s Melissa Yang in 2022. "But I believe in my heart that there's another way. You can find flow and you can be at ease on the field and you can have bliss when you play. I felt like, in order for me to get closer to the player and athlete I wanted to be, I had to take a step back and focus on how close I can get to that blissful space off the field as a human and really understand my identity as a full person outside of an athlete."[29] (Of course, the NWSL is far from the only league that must continue to reckon with mistreatment of its athletes—it's just been a particularly prominent example in recent years.)

There aren't any easy answers for supporting athletes' mental health in the long term. Coaches, teams, and leagues can do more and more, but not one of those steps is a magic bullet. "Anybody that sells you a quick fix for mental health is lying to you," Love said. It all comes down to the athletes themselves, too. Speaking from his own experience, he added, "You have to be consistent. You have to do the work. It's not always going to be easy. Even for me, when I first started going to therapy, it got a lot worse before it got better. But on the other side of it, there's so much happiness—which is a moving target, mind you—but there's so much to be had on the other side of it."

*　*　*

The movement DeRozan and Love sparked within sports was truly groundbreaking. As it unfolded over the next couple of years, we saw leagues and teams slowly up their games—a process that's continued to this day in leagues like the NWSL. We saw a largely empathetic audience in and out of sports ready to receive and start to process such powerful information and the emotion behind it.

It seemed like the door—the stubborn, ever-present barrier that prevented high-profile athletes from opening up publicly—had been Kool-Aid-manned straight through. As we'd find out in the years afterward, the door was, in the grand scheme of things, perhaps only ajar, which is not to downplay the significance of athletes like DeRozan and Love but only to acknowledge further progress on the horizon: The coronavirus pandemic, which would begin in earnest in the United States in March 2020, was still to come.

With the pandemic, along with our physical health, our mental health—whether or not we were athletes—would also be thrown into disarray, especially during the early months of lockdown. As big as DeRozan's and Love's celebrities were (and still are), they would be followed in speaking out by superstars on the global stage, people whose careers were thrown off course due to their own mental health. With the extenuating circumstances we were all living through, those messages took on even more import. When Naomi Osaka and Simone Biles spoke up, they stunned the world.

CHAPTER 6

The Greats Chime In

Anxiety and Depression amid a Pandemic

PRESS CONFERENCES AREN'T EASY. FOR AN EXAMPLE OF HOW ATHLETES get pelted with question after question by near strangers after a crushing loss, look no further than Naomi Osaka's experiences. Let's examine the tennis star's September 2019 press conference, in particular, which took place after she lost in the fourth round of the U.S. Open; certainly, for an athlete of her status, anything less than a win at a major can be a disappointing result. Before leaving the complex—but, blessedly for her, in this case after taking a shower, she was sure to note—Osaka had to answer for her play. After all, she was the tournament's defending champion. The following, for reference, is from a press conference in which Osaka at one point described herself as "more chill."[1]

Right off the bat, the No. 1 seed was asked what made the difference in the two-set (7–5, 6–4) match, which she dropped to No. 13 Belinda Bencic. "I think she played pretty clean," Osaka responded. She added, "I don't want to answer like, saying that, like, everything I did wrong, you know? Like, I want to think about it more positively."

She was then asked about her knee. She downplayed the ailment and explicitly chose to not blame it for her loss. "I just needed to take a pain-killer," she said. Next came a question about whether she walked away from the match with a greater sense of sportsmanship. A gimme. Osaka, in part, said, "Yeah, for me, right now I have this feeling of sadness, but

97

I also feel like I have learned so much during this tournament. Honestly, of course I wanted to defend this tournament."

Then came a question about whether Osaka's sadness on that day was different than her sadness after other recent major losses. And so on and so forth. Then she answered questions from Japanese media. Near the end of the ordeal, she finally said, in English, what's on her mind: "To be honest, I'm not even thinking about playing tennis there right now. All I'm thinking about is, like, the takoyaki [a Japanese snack with diced octopus]." On that note, she was free.

Osaka seemed lighthearted enough at that particular press conference, often smiling as she offered up answers, including one in which she praised Russian men's player Daniil Medvedev's sarcasm. But even on a relatively good day, she was tasked with describing why her performance faltered, her current and past moments of sadness, and what was ailing her—on a day that she, in some minds, failed at her job. It's a lot to handle.

* * *

Nearly two years later, in May 2021, despite its being a requirement of her job, Osaka declined to participate in French Open press conferences. She never wanted to be a distraction. Although it wasn't entirely clear to some critics at first, her goal was just to protect her mental health. "I've often felt that people have no regard for athletes [*sic*] mental health, and this rings very true whenever I see a press conference or partake in one," the four-time Grand Slam champion wrote on Instagram in a post that's no longer available. "We're often sat there and asked questions that we've been asked multiple times before or asked questions that bring doubt into our minds and I'm just not going to subject myself to people that doubt me."[2]

Osaka had never advanced past the third round at Roland Garros. It's widely known that clay is her worst surface—and it's something reporters constantly harp on as they pepper her with questions. Her decision evoked memories of Marshawn Lynch, the Seattle Seahawks player infamous for telling the media a whopping 29 times during Super Bowl media day in 2015, "I'm here so I don't get fined."[3] Lynch may have also been protecting his mental health, but he never mentioned it if so.

"Girl, do you," one of Osaka's role models, Serena Williams, commented on her Instagram post. "Your life is yours to live!"[4] The French Tennis Federation, apparently, did not feel similarly. It threatened to fine Osaka and later threatened to increase the penalty amount, in addition to expelling her from the tournament, should she not meet with the media. "If the organizations think that they can just keep saying, 'Do press or you're gonna be fined,' and continue to ignore the mental health of the athletes that are at the centerpiece of their [corporation], then I just gotta laugh," Osaka wrote in her initial post.[5]

The pushback to Osaka's decision was for the most part polite, but it was also swift. "While it's important that everyone has the right to speak their truth, I have always believed that as professional athletes we have a responsibility to make ourselves available to the media," tweeted tennis legend Billie Jean King, in part.[6] Men's star Rafael Nadal of Spain echoed a similar thought about the importance of the media. "I understand her, but on the other hand, for me, I mean, without the press, without the people who normally travel, who are writing the news and achievements that we are having around the world, we probably will not be the athletes that we are today," he said. Then–world No. 1 Ash Barty didn't comment on Osaka (then No. 2) specifically but said, in general, "We know what we sign up for as professional tennis players."[7]

Then there were relentless critics like Piers Morgan, who, unsurprisingly, didn't bother with niceties, calling Osaka an "arrogant spoiled brat whose fame and fortune appears to have inflated her ego to gigantic proportions" in his *Daily Mail* column.[8] Fellow conservative pundits Clay Travis and Megyn Kelly later weighed in, too, calling out Osaka for posing for magazine covers after saying she didn't want to deal with the press. Not that it matters, but the covers were shot well before Osaka's mental health break.

* * *

The situation between Osaka and French Open officials soon deteriorated even further. She gave a brief on-court interview after beating Romania's Patricia Maria Tig in the tournament's first round but did not sit for a news conference. ("I'd say it is a work in progress," Osaka said when asked about her clay game. "Hopefully the more I play the better I get."[9]) True to their word, the officials fined her $15,000. She ultimately withdrew from the event in Paris altogether, citing her desire to return the focus to the actual tennis being played by her colleagues.

In announcing her withdrawal, Osaka posted a second message to Instagram. This one was deeper, more personal. "I would never trivialize mental health or use the term lightly," she wrote. "The truth is that I have suffered long bouts of depression since the U.S. Open in 2018 and I have had a really hard time coping with that."[10] The U.S. Open that September, it seemed, was likely a traumatic experience for both her and Williams, her opponent in the final. During the match, Williams received a code violation for apparently receiving coaching (which is not allowed during tennis matches and which she denied had happened). She then got frustrated with officiating, smashing her racket. After an argument with the official, she got hit with a verbal abuse code violation. She automatically lost an entire game as a result. Osaka was the better player through the chaos, yet she cried during the trophy ceremony as boos rained down on her from the crowd. Williams cried, too.

Osaka called bowing out of French Open press conferences "self-care." In a joint statement, tennis officials from all four Grand Slam countries preferred to see it as "an unfair advantage." It's clear the world's highest-paid female tennis player didn't necessarily *want* to go into depth on her mental health struggles. And why should she have had to? A brief nod to the issue or even some "personal reasons" should've been enough. Instead, Osaka felt she had to go into more detail, withdraw from the tournament, and take a step back from tennis to gather herself.

Some of those who had criticized Osaka changed their tune after learning more about her reasoning for wanting to sit out press conferences. King tweeted, "It's incredibly brave that Naomi Osaka has revealed her truth about her struggle with depression. Right now, the important thing is that we give her the space and time she needs. We wish her well."[11]

Alex Abad-Santos, writing for *Vox*, couldn't help but notice a curious discrepancy between Osaka's withdrawal and another famous player's withdrawal from the same major the same year. "In the days following Osaka's French Open departure, Roger Federer bowed out June 6, citing his health," Abad-Santos wrote. "There was no pushback or demand for more information from the French Tennis Federation or the media. Federer was, quite simply, looking out for his own well-being. He said he needed to listen to his body. Everyone believed him."[12]

Federer was recovering from two knee surgeries. Funny how he wasn't met with any vitriol for his choice—as a society, we tend to trust physical injuries, many of which are outwardly visible, more than mental distress, which is easier to write off as imaginary, no matter how real it may be. It probably also didn't hurt that Federer is a white man, which inherently makes him more trustworthy in the eyes of many. Mental illness—or even smaller moments of mental ill health in an otherwise "healthy" brain—is very real. Osaka should have been given the benefit of the doubt, as every athlete should. She was just listening to her body.

* * *

Naomi Osaka, along with gymnastics GOAT (perhaps even overall GOAT) Simone Biles a few months later, drastically altered the landscape around athletes' disclosures of mental health issues in the eyes of other athletes and experts alike. Almost every one of the nearly 100 people I spoke to for this book cited at least one—most often both—of their influences on the ongoing dialogue and shifting attitudes toward athletes and their needs. Before we go any further, let's establish this: Neither Biles nor Osaka likely set out to be heroes for the masses; on an individual level, they were simply making decisions that were best for their minds and bodies. (In fact, Osaka told Morgan Jerkins in *Self* that seeing the reaction to her openness and the athletes who followed in her footsteps was "a bit strange."[13]) But women of their stature disclosing—from a place of strength—issues that have historically been perceived as weaknesses empowers others in sports to do the same.

"As a Black woman, I'm proud of Naomi for sharing that. Because I went through challenges, but at the same time, we've been taught to give a quick nod if you're able to give a quick nod and then push through," said Akilah Carter-Francique, former executive director of the Institute for the Study of Sport, Society, and Social Change and a professor of African American studies at San José State University.

DiDi Richards, a former guard for the New York Liberty, said she can draw a direct line between Biles's and Osaka's disclosures and her own mental health advocacy. Richards dealt with anxiety while playing for Baylor University and openly wanted to be drafted by the Liberty because of the emphasis she felt they placed on mental wellness. "Because Naomi is comfortable talking about it, then I'm comfortable now talking about it," she told me. "I hope I can be that for someone." She likely is that person for someone already or will be one day soon: Today, speaking out in the WNBA is increasingly common. In addition to Biles and Osaka, Richards credits her own openness to Katie Lou Samuelson, a forward in the league drafted two years before Richards. As we've seen before, mental health disclosures can be chain reactions.

The COVID-19 pandemic, during which both Osaka and Biles spoke out about their mental health and stepped away from their sports, however briefly, kicked that chain reaction along even further. In fact, Biles had told me for *Sports Illustrated* more than a year before the postponed Tokyo Olympics that she, like other elite athletes, had been struggling with her mental health since learning the Games were pushed back due to the pandemic.

In a 2022 literature review in the *American Journal of Sports Medicine*, 32 of the 35 studies analyzed associated the pandemic with poor mental health outcomes for athletes, especially for female athletes and athletes competing at elite levels. One 2020 study reviewed, from the *International Journal of Environmental Research and Public Health*, found that across elite athletes in three sports in Sweden (handball, soccer, and ice hockey), 66 percent were worried about the future of their sports and 51 percent about *their* future in sports. More than a year is a long time to shave off at a high level in the business, where people are often described as being on the "wrong side" of 30.

Many athletes lost access to not only their sports and training facilities while quarantining, but also the in-person mental health care they may have been accustomed to. On top of that, some athletes, depending on their economic backgrounds, might not have had the means or resources to benefit from telehealth care from therapists or psychiatrists. Or they might have had the above but not a private space from which to chat candidly. And for those experiencing conditions like suicidal ideation, the onset of psychosis, or an eating disorder, remote care simply may not be adequate treatment. These athletes weren't just losing a recreational activity or garden-variety exercise; they were losing their livelihoods, in some cases the only way they knew how to provide for themselves. They were left to wonder whether that livelihood would ever come back. So the pandemic exacerbated the mental health crisis for everyone—but these effects were outsized for athletes.

* * *

The most decorated gymnast of all time arrived in Tokyo after five years of training, up from the usual four. Simone Biles, 24, was coming off the 2016 Games in Rio, where she'd made U.S. Olympic history by winning five medals—four of them gold. The years in between those two Games were not uneventful.

In 2018, more than a year after the *Indianapolis Star* broke the news about the sexually abusive USA Gymnastics team doctor Larry Nassar, Biles said that she, too, along with McKayla Maroney and more than 150 other gymnasts, had been sexually assaulted by him. "Most of you know me as a happy, giggly, and energetic girl," she began her Twitter statement that January. "But lately . . . I've felt a bit broken and the more I try to shut off the voice in my head the louder it screams. I am not afraid to tell my story anymore." The post was hashtagged #MeToo.[14]

By the end of 2018, almost a year after that disclosure, Biles had told *Good Morning America* that she takes anxiety medication and regularly sees a therapist. Those disclosures would not be her last about the state of her mental health. For Biles, it seems to be an ongoing process. "The scars of this horrific abuse continue to live with all of us," she testified before the Senate Judiciary Committee about Nassar in September 2021, following the Tokyo Games.[15]

Although she didn't appear to talk publicly about Nassar while in Tokyo, the scars Biles has were arguably evident there, as she fought to preserve her mental and physical health. She felt at the Olympics that her coaches' words of encouragement weren't resonating with her like they usually did. "I got more and more nervous," she later told Camonghne Felix for *The Cut*. "I didn't feel as confident as I should have been with as much training as we had."[16]

Then her anxiety started manifesting itself physically. Between the preliminaries and the team final, Biles experienced trouble performing. First, she got lost in the air practicing a floor routine. She wrote it off as a fluke and tried again the next day, leading up to the team finals, and again she faltered. "I just could not get a sense of where I was in the air," she later told NBC.[17]

Biles at first tried to press on, competing in vault on the opening rotation of the team finals. (Incidentally, that was July 27, 2021, the same day Osaka was ousted from her Olympic tournament in the third round to Czechia's Markéta Vondroušová.) She landed low in her first attempt. What was supposed to be a Yurchenko 2½ (also called an Amanar, for Romanian gymnast Simona Amanar) became a less difficult Yurchenko 1½. (This vault, named after former Soviet gymnast Natalia Yurchenko, entails a roundoff onto the springboard and a back handspring onto the vaulting table. The number is indicative of how many twists are involved.) Following the vault, Biles sat with her doctor, left the arena, and then returned to announce to her teammates she had withdrawn from the meet. USA Gymnastics released a statement attributing her withdrawal to a medical issue. Biles proceeded to cheer relentlessly for her teammates—Suni Lee, Jordan Chiles, and Grace McCallum—who nabbed silver in the team finals behind the Russia Olympic Committee.

"I have to focus on my mental health and not jeopardize my health and well-being," Biles said that day. "It just sucks when you're fighting with your own head."[18] USA Gymnastics as a whole took a mental rest day following the team finals. Biles would then be evaluated every day to see whether she would be able to take part in the individual all-around and other events.

Then Biles withdrew from the individual all-around final, which was to take place the following day. She had won gold in the event in Rio in 2016. "The outpouring love & support I've received has made me realize I'm more than my accomplishments and gymnastics which I never truly believed before," she tweeted with a white heart emoji.[19] On the day of the individual all-around final, Biles spoke up again. "For anyone saying I quit. I didn't quit, my mind & body are simply not in sync," she wrote in an Instagram story. Biles shared clips of her training from that morning. In one, she dismounts from the uneven bars and lands, into heavy padding, on her back—one and a half twists shy of what she said she should've executed.[20]

The same day as the individual all-around final, Biles, via an Instagram story, introduced the non-gymnast world to the frightening concept of the "twisties." Sports Illustrated baseball writer Stephanie Apstein, who covered the Tokyo Games, aptly described the predicament a few days later as "a form of gymnastics yips that leaves its sufferers feeling lost in the air."[21] It's possible to twist when you hadn't planned to or not twist in the proper way or as much as you had planned to. As a result, you can land on parts of your body that are not meant to be landed on. "My perspective has never changed so quickly from wanting to be on a podium to wanting to be able to go home, by myself, without any crutches," Biles later told Felix.[22] It's not hyperbole to say the twisties are a matter of life and death.

One day after explaining the twisties to the masses, Biles withdrew from the vault and bars finals. The following day, she withdrew from the floor final as well. As she sat out these events, Biles didn't shirk the spotlight or step back from her role in supporting her teammates. Instead, she was in the stands loudly cheering on Team USA, including those who had replaced her on various apparatuses. Then, at last, some good news came from Biles: She would make her comeback in the last event of the meet—the balance beam final. To get to the point of competing, Biles had to be cleared by a Team USA sport psychologist and medical doctors. She had never imagined she would be. She also altered her balance beam routine to make the dismount easier: Instead of a twist, she completed a double pike, which is so simple that she hadn't done it in competition since age 12. It "just meant the world to be back out there," she told reporters.[23]

But Biles wasn't *just* back out there. She earned bronze on beam, her seventh career Olympic medal. It meant more to her, she said, than all her golds. "I've pushed through so much the last five years and the last week while I've even been here," Biles told Hota Kotb on *Today*. "It was very emotional, and I'm just proud of myself."[24]

* * *

As with Osaka's, Biles's critics—largely from the political right—were loud. "Simone got an incredible amount of backlash, as if she wanted to be struggling on the world stage," said Gracie Gold, an Olympic figure skater who helped the U.S. team win a bronze medal in Sochi in 2014. "As if that's something we all dream of."

Conservative pundit Charlie Kirk declared, "We are raising a generation of weak people like Simone Biles." He also called her a "selfish sociopath" and a "shame to the country."[25] Fox personalities derided her, too. She was "the biggest quitter in sports," according to Ben Maller,[26] and Doug Gottlieb claimed she hadn't faced criticism in her career (a laughable idea). The deputy attorney general from Texas at the time, Aaron Reitz, called her a "national embarrassment."[27] (He later deleted his tweet and apologized.) Jemele Hill, writing for *The Atlantic*, eviscerated Biles's critics. "Some people—conservative men in particular," she wrote, "simply cannot bear to see a woman of color making her own choices about what's best for her."[28]

As loud as Biles's detractors may have been, her supporters were seemingly a far bigger contingent. Fellow Olympic legend Michael Phelps, for one, was eager to contextualize the meaning of her disclosure of mental health struggles. "I hope this is an opportunity for us to jump on board and to even blow this mental health thing even more wide open," he told NBC's Mike Tirico on prime-time coverage during the Games.[29]

Those adding to the chorus were other athletes, along with politicians and performers. "WE LOVE YOU," tweeted former Olympic figure skater Adam Rippon.[30] U.S. Representative Alexandria Ocasio-Cortez, a Democrat from New York, told *TMZ*, "What Simone Biles did in these Olympics, she showed that she's a role model not just as an athlete but a leader for just all people."[31] Pop star Justin Bieber, who has been open about his own mental health, wrote on Instagram, "Sometimes our no's are more powerful than our yes's. When what you normally love starts to steal your joy it's important we take a step back to evaluate why."[32]

Step back Biles did. She didn't really have a choice, physically, if she wanted to ensure she would live. Her body was telling her she needed a mental break, and she listened. All she had endured each day in the lead-up to Tokyo was made clear as she testified in September 2021 against Nassar: "As a recent competitor in the Tokyo Games who was a survivor of this horror, I can assure you the impacts of this man's abuse are not over or ever forgotten. The announcement in the spring of 2020 that the Tokyo Games were to be postponed for a year meant that I would be going to the gym, to training, to therapy, living daily among the reminders of this story for another 365 days."[33] Her body and mind apparently didn't falter during that year, but it's no surprise that they did eventually given all the weight they were bearing.

* * *

At the same time Biles was wrestling with the twisties and deciding whether she felt she could safely push through, another Olympic athlete, in a different sport, was dealing with her own issues—also physical and mental. In women's soccer, Canadian national team goalkeeper Stephanie Labbé would go on to win the gold medal with her teammates. But her path through the Games, like Biles's, was anything but direct.

Early in the second half of Canada's opening game of the tournament, against Japan, Labbé challenged an attacker for the ball and sustained a rib joint injury. She stayed in to stop a penalty kick but was medically ruled out for the remainder of the match—and for the entirety of Canada's next contest, against Chile. She was told by her doctors that it wasn't a situation where she could simply push through the pain she was in and play, that it could be destructive to her health.

Labbé got the all clear six days after the injury, though, and returned to the tournament in Canada's last group-stage game, versus Great Britain. A draw in that match was enough to vault Canada to the knockout rounds. In the quarterfinal, Labbé and company beat Brazil 4–3 on penalty kicks, with Labbé making two key saves. "That game was the peak of it all," she reflected to me months after the Games, shortly before she retired. "This positive adrenaline rush, this peak of emotion. And you know, my phone blowing up after. . . . I just wasn't able to come down from that high."

From that point in the tournament on, with about a week to go, Labbé couldn't train in Tokyo. In fact, she couldn't do much of anything besides lay down in her dark room with her eyes closed, listening to her heart beat out of her chest. She couldn't control her breathing. She talked to her personal sport psychologist once or twice every day toward the end of the tournament. But somehow she showed up on the pitch come game time in the semifinal and then, a few days later, the gold-medal match. "The athlete Stephanie Labbé was in a great space," she said. "It was the human Stephanie Labbé that wasn't."

Labbé had been through anxiety and depression before. She had been candid about her difficult comedown after the 2016 Rio Games, during which she earned a bronze medal for her country. She was also candid with me near the start of the pandemic about how the crisis was affecting her in terms of mental health and what she and her partner, Olympic cyclist and skier Georgia Simmerling, were doing to keep their minds intact.

Behind Labbé's strong play in Tokyo, Canada went on to beat the United States in the Tokyo semifinals and then Sweden in the final. It would be a month before she felt well enough mentally to acknowledge the triumph, even to herself. "Just the thought of the Olympics brought me into the heightened anxiety state," she said. After weeks of not wanting to talk about the Games, one day, in a hotel room in Paris, where

Labbé was staying before finding an apartment for her new club gig, she finally put on her medal and cracked open a beer. She texted Simmerling a picture to celebrate.

Naturally, Labbé can't help but compare and contrast what she went through with what Biles did because of the timing of the Olympics. "I think about the amount of people that were like, 'Oh, all of a sudden the day before [Biles] just can't compete,'" Labbé said. "It's not recognizing how something can actually affect you. For her, it was a totally different experience than for me, for example, when I was able to step on the field and disassociate from it. But in her sport, it was actually very dangerous for her to go in and not be fully confident."

Seeing an international superstar come forward represented quite a drastic shift in the landscape around athlete mental health from where it was even a decade ago, Labbé said. "Talking about mental health, you'd be afraid that you're weak or maybe a coach wouldn't select you or wouldn't play you because you have mental health challenges, and maybe that means if the game gets really hard, you won't be able to cope with it. Or, are you mentally strong enough?" Labbé said. "Now I think the conversation's turning to where we're not seeing it as a weakness. We're actually seeing it as a strength."

* * *

The ripple effects of Osaka's and Biles's openness are everywhere, extending far beyond just Labbé and her peers. Like those who came before these athletes in disclosing mental health struggles and mental illnesses, they are changing the game. Only this time, it's on the biggest scale to date.

Bianca Andreescu is one such prominent athlete who followed in Osaka's and Biles's footsteps during the pandemic. In March 2020, the tennis star made a bet with a friend who thought COVID-19 would last three months. Andreescu thought it would last just six weeks. The pandemic, of course, would last far longer and be far more grueling than most thought. During the early period in Canada, she couldn't train or even see her family and friends.

The 2019 U.S. Open champion (who told me on asking where I live that she loves Queens—wonder why!) announced a mental health break from tennis in December 2021, explaining that she would skip the next Australian Open. The Romanian Canadian player said that she had been off her game both physically and mentally since her grandmother spent weeks in an intensive care unit in Romania with COVID-19 and that she herself had to quarantine for weeks due to a positive test. "A lot of days, I did not feel like myself, especially while I was training and/or playing matches," she had tweeted.[34] She didn't exactly see herself as depressed, she later told me, but she thinks she would've gotten to that point had she not taken a break. "When I am going through something, I just say I'm going through something," she said. "I don't like to put a label on anything because then . . . it truly becomes real."

Tennis, to Andreescu, had stopped being an outlet to relieve stress, she told me. One major factor was that over time, she had begun to feel more of the pressure of the off-court obligations of being a premier player on the tour. "I love[d] my private life," she said. "I don't have it anymore, sadly. Obviously, with becoming a brand, you don't really have a private life." That feeling is not unique to tennis, but it can be amplified in individual sports because there are no teammates to share the tougher moments with: of getting support in your training, of dealing with the press after a big loss, and of looking and acting your best at all times for sponsors. The tennis machine takes very young players—often teenagers—and transforms them into brands, whether they like it or not.

Talking to Andreescu six weeks after she made her decision public (she had considered it for two months beforehand but was apprehensive due to the reaction she'd draw), she stood by it as the right call. "I'm like, look, I really have to step back because I cannot continue like this," she said. "I can't continue to put the people that I love through this. Because whatever affects me affects them as well because they truly care about me and vice versa. So that was really hard, and it took a lot of courage." She also referred to herself, Osaka, and Biles as "outsiders" who face pushback from their still-uncommon choices as elite athletes to skip competitions.

"Us athletes, when we grow up and we train to become who we want to become, we're taught to just push through everything," Andreescu said.

"Even if you're injured, just keep pushing. But I learned that you really need to know your limits."

One of her sport's all-time greats, Billie Jean King, who at first had a negative knee-jerk reaction to Osaka's decision to step back from press conferences (before coming around and supporting her), reassured Andreescu and told her to trust herself. "I remember I was just having a tough time stepping on the court," Andreescu said. "She's like, 'It's normal. Don't beat yourself up about it.'" King also told Andreescu to stop playing tennis when it stops making her happy. Andreescu, for her part, said that she took the break because tennis usually does make her happy and that she wants to preserve that feeling and be an example for others—just like Biles and Osaka were examples for her.

* * *

U.S. Olympic gold medalist snowboarder Chloe Kim didn't start going to therapy until around the time of the Tokyo Summer Games. She also started speaking out about her mental health. "I think I was more open about it because of Simone and Naomi, especially, just seeing how they were so outspoken about the mental health problems that they were dealing with and how that's never talked about within professional athletics whatsoever," she said. She also called Biles and Osaka "amazing goddesses" who have inspired her.

A few years back, right after the PyeongChang Winter Olympics in 2018, Kim was not formally diagnosed with depression, but she said if that wasn't an accurate descriptor, it was "pretty damn close." She was just 17. "I got lost," she said. "I felt like I had no purpose in life." Her yearlong break from snowboarding after those Games to start college was always the plan, even before she started to struggle. "I had accomplished my purpose in life. When that's gone, you kind of spiral . . . and you lose your sense of being. That was really hard for me to deal with because I went from the craziest, most hectic two years leading into the Olympics to just nothing," she added.

Kim attended Princeton but returned to snowboarding once COVID-19 hit. The pandemic, having originated in China, also led to a huge spike in anti-Asian violence, and that weighed on her, too. (Kim is Korean American.) She decided to take another season off after the 2022 Beijing Games. "Now's the time for me to be Chloe the person, not the snowboarder," she said. When we spoke in April 2022, she planned to use her time off to pursue fashion design or maybe acting. She also just wanted to enjoy being 21. As for the conversation around mental health and mental illness that she's become a part of, she wants to see more people understand that the likes of Biles and Osaka aren't necessarily done competing, like their critics want you to believe. "It's just you have a bad day," Kim said. "You're struggling, and that's okay."

In the last couple of years alone, mental health support in the United States and a handful of other countries for Olympians and Paralympians has increased drastically. In September 2020, the USOPC hired Jessica Bartley, a clinical associate professor at the University of Denver, as its first director of mental health services. Bartley is a former athlete herself. About 20 years ago, the aggressive, five-foot-five goalie planned to play soccer at the University of Texas, but injuries derailed her career. "There just weren't a lot of mental health resources, and so I wanted to be the resource that I didn't have as an athlete—especially as an elite athlete," Bartley said.

One of the first moves Bartley oversaw at the USOPC was the creation of a crisis hotline for athletes, staffed 24/7. Next came a 60-page emergency action plan for the national governing bodies that oversee each sport. It addresses whom to call and what to look for when a mental health emergency arises. It covers a wide range of conditions, including anxiety, depression, substance use, and eating disorders. There's also a registry for athletes to use; through it, they can access almost 200 licensed mental health providers nationwide who apply with at least five years of experience in elite sports.

Bartley also said there are now small support groups for athletes to come together and share experiences, including athletes who didn't ultimately qualify for the Games. It's about eight to 12 athletes per group, along with a facilitator. There are "pivot groups," which are designed for athletes who are retiring to get emotional support and education.

Parenting and motherhood have been the focus of other support groups, and there have been dedicated groups for athletes of color.

The USOPC's health insurance covers 100 percent of mental health–related costs—no copays, deductibles, or session limits. The organization can also cover care for up to two years after an athlete's retirement. Near the end of 2021, Bartley said, the USOPC also created a mental health assistance fund for Team USA athletes not on the organization's insurance. The donor-funded initiative covers everything from an ADHD evaluation to costs for an athlete who may have gotten kicked off insurance due to a suspension to treatment for a retired athlete.

Bartley said her team pays attention to callouts of U.S. Olympic mental health culture, like HBO's *The Weight of Gold*, the 2020 Phelps-narrated documentary that shines a light on the occasionally deadly mental illness experienced by Olympians. It strongly asserts that the USOPC hasn't done enough to take care of its elite athletes. Bartley's crew listens to try to understand athletes' concerns and fill in holes in coverage. At the same time, she thinks the USOPC offerings have come a long way in recent years. "If someone says, 'Hey, we don't have resources,' I'm like, 'Actually, this insurance is incredible,'" she said.

Bartley also runs a mental health task force, started early in 2020, before COVID-19 and before she came aboard. The group meets monthly and features athletes, former athletes, coaches, and mental health professionals. Perhaps the most interesting part of what Bartley does is to share what might be thought of as competitive secrets with her counterparts in Australia, Canada, Denmark, and the United Kingdom. Some of those countries have universal mental health care and don't face the same challenges the United States does. But, for example, Team Canada does a separate assessment alongside each sport's national governing body and lets Bartley sit in on the process so she could plan to do something similar with the USOPC.

"That's one of the things on the horizon of like, 'Okay, we've built out some really basic services in mental health, we have these ideas, but what do we do sport to sport that could look a little bit different?'" Bartley said. "And that's what I think this needs assessment would really show us. And—I hate to say it—it's just kind of nice to just borrow it from Canada."

* * *

Make no mistake: There's still a long way to go when it comes to getting our top athletes the care they need, and not everyone feels that the USOPC progress Bartley spoke of is enough. Phelps told me so when we spoke in 2022 for *Sports Illustrated*. "[The USOPC] says they're offering [support], but they're not offering anything," he said. "I want people to actually do something. The sport psychologists and all these different groups of people that they have hired, we don't feel safe and comfortable going to them. So we don't go to them, and then they still don't understand why we don't go to them. So there's some kind of disconnect."[35]

And remember Osaka's trouble with press conferences? She rejoined the tour later in 2021, but it's not like journalists, mental health professionals, or athletes themselves have found a way to make press conferences a healthier experience that still gives reporters the access they—and readers and viewers—need. Osaka raised one idea in *Time*, which I think is a good one: "My No. 1 suggestion would be to allow a small number of 'sick days' per year where you are excused from your press commitments without having to disclose your personal reasons. I believe this would bring sport in line with the rest of society."[36] But when I spoke to journalists and mental health experts for a potential *Sports Illustrated* story on what could be changed, my sources were mostly at a loss. I never wrote the piece.

Osaka's life on the tour has been anything but seamless since her break. At Indian Wells in March 2022, a fan heckled her during her second-round match against Veronika Kudermetova. Osaka lost and addressed the crowd (an unusual move): "To be honest, I've gotten heckled before. It didn't really bother me," she said. "But [being] heckled here, I watched a video of Venus and Serena getting heckled here, and if you've never watched it, you should watch it. I don't know why, but it went into my head, and it got replayed a lot. I'm trying not to cry."[37] (Famously, the Williams sisters and their father, Richard, were heckled at the tournament in 2001 and accused of match fixing before Venus withdrew from a semifinal match. Richard said people called him the N-word.)

The incident with Osaka caused *Sports Illustrated*'s L. Jon Wertheim to wonder whether she should be competing at all. "She has made the point that just because an injury doesn't show up on an X-ray or MRI doesn't make it less real," he wrote. "And she's right. But by the same logic, the same way an athlete with a bad back or an unhealed knee might not be able to compete, it seems fair and reasonable to ask whether Osaka could use more time away to find answers for herself."[38] After Indian Wells, Osaka attended therapy on a consistent basis for the first time.

And yet people without Osaka's status may not even feel comfortable or financially able to make the choice to step away from sports and seek additional help. It's an option currently afforded only to established, privileged players, and that needs to change. But how? It's sort of like those pesky press conferences but on a much larger scale: Only some people agree that mental health care for athletes needs improving, and not many of those people seem to have a clue as to how to make it better. Money is, as usual, probably the answer (or at least a big part of the answer): Pay athletes more, give them better health care, and see them as people first and not as brands to be maintained. And it's not just professional and Olympic athletes we need to ask these questions and make these seismic changes on behalf of, either. At the college level, athletes often have even fewer resources and, obviously, a whole lot less money. But they experience mental illness all the same.

CHAPTER 7

On Campus

The Push for Better Care at Colleges

BY THE TIME RECEIVER GABE MARKS GOT TO WASHINGTON STATE TO play football in 2012, he was overwhelmed. "You become a star in your field, and you're getting recruited in high school and dealing with the pressures of that," he said. "And then that pressure just mounts, and by the time you are in college, playing at a Division I school in a prestigious conference and the school is banking billions of dollars. . . . The coaches are getting paid a billion dollars a year, and they got families. Suddenly you are responsible for the lives of grown men keeping their jobs and whatnot." That's a lot for an 18-year-old to manage.

Marks played for Washington State until 2016. He didn't get drafted into the NFL the next year but ultimately signed as a free agent with the New York Jets, projecting as a slot receiver. Then he got waived. "There was nobody that I felt comfortable to talk to at the time about it," he later told the *Seattle Times*.[1] Left without adequate tools to transition to the real world, Marks felt lost. "It was a harrowing process," he told me in the spring of 2022. "A lot of death and rebirth happening. It constantly felt like every day I was like a new child born into the world, really. It was hard." Marks stressed that his situation is not abnormal. Most athletes around his age are left wondering what their next step will be, what their new career will be. "We all leave [sports] sooner than we'd like, unless you're Tom Brady or one of those very fortunate few."

Marks has used his time away from sports to pursue a new profession: psychology. He's a therapist at Thrive Health and Collective Wellness, a company his aunt runs in Marina del Rey, California. He thinks about getting a PhD one day. "I wanted to see what was going on with people and start to understand the patterns that we all share in terms of our lives in this particular society," he said. "Hopefully I can work within other cultures and other societies. Everyone has their different way of viewing the world based on the world view that they have, but in our Western society, I was very interested to see what made people tick, so that led me down the path of doing the clinical work."

He doesn't work with college athlete or former athlete populations—yet. He wants to because he knows acutely what they have been through as someone who's played through anxiety and stress himself. "What's going on with your team?" he asked, thinking through how he'd approach working alongside one. "How many anxious players do you have? How many players do you have that are experiencing depression? . . . How many players are experiencing arrested development or dealing with trauma that's unresolved? How can these things, if discussed and worked through in a treatment plan and therapy, allow your team to succeed even more?"

* * *

The mental health care available for collegiate athletes like Marks has improved drastically in recent years. "I think the changes have been pretty dramatic from 2007 and even five years before that, when I was an athlete and coaching," said Ian Connole, a Dartmouth senior associate athletic director for the Peak Performance program, which offers the Ivy League school's athletes a holistic approach to physical, intellectual, and personal growth. He graduated in 2006 from Division III Skidmore, where he played basketball. "It's been a slowly increasing open dialogue. I haven't seen a floodgate moment or one watershed event but much more a steady incline in professionals available, administrators noticing the need and actually creating positions to hire for that, and student-athletes and athletes broadly talking about the mental side of sport."

Some of the changes have come from the top. Brian Hainline, the NCAA's chief medical officer since 2013, has made mental health a main concern, if not *the* main concern. Just one week into the job, Hainline, a neurologist, met with collegiate athletes from advisory committees across Divisions I, II, and III as part of the annual NCAA convention. He said the leaders from each conference independently asked him, "Can you please make mental health your priority?" Ahead of even concussions, they felt it was an issue requiring his immediate attention. "I pledged to them that that would be our priority," Hainline said. Within a year, he had formed a working group. "I knew [mental health] was a deal. The student-athletes told me, 'Look, please make this the *biggest* deal.'"

The NCAA, then, in 2016, put out a 40-page guide of mental health best practices for its more than 1,100 member institutions. It was endorsed by 24 leading mental health, medical, and sports medicine organizations nationwide. The guide included recommendations for schools on having clinical practitioners available to offer mental health care, procedures for referring athletes to qualified practitioners, pre-participation mental health screenings for athletes, and the cultivation of athletics environments that support mental well-being. Each division responded by passing legislation that said every school should have mental health programs in line with the recommendations of the best practices document. While not binding and not perfect (on one page, the NCAA recommends local police officers as a resource for helping struggling students), the moves marked a step in the right direction.

Another of the steps needed: "How can all of their very good recommendations be implemented?" asked Claudia Reardon, a sport psychiatrist and professor at the University of Wisconsin. "And how can institutions be compelled to put resources toward mental health when, of course, money is in short supply and, quite honestly, licensed mental health providers are in short supply?" It's a good question that hasn't been resolved.

In addition to publishing best practices, Hainline also tackled the NCAA's mental health issue by equipping coaches, who he considers to be data driven, with information. Mental health symptoms and disorders, he said, have the potential to predict recovery timelines from physical injuries. "If you have a physical injury and you develop, say, depression or anxiety post-injury, that's going to delay your recovery, and mental symptoms and disorders can negatively impact performance," he said. "When coaches see that there are data that say, 'Look, our athlete's not gonna be performing as well and may be more injured, or their injury may be more prolonged,' they will listen to that." It might be a cynical way of looking at the situation, and you might say coaches should care about athletes' well-being for non–performance-related reasons first and foremost, but at the same time, it's clear that Hainline will take the win whichever way he can get it.

Despite Hainline's progress on multiple fronts, he acknowledged in our conversation in late 2021, "The room for improvement is astronomical." It's hard not to agree. Only 69 percent of female athletes and 63 percent of male athletes (out of more than 9,800 surveyed by the NCAA) even know where to go on campus if they have mental health issues. And less than half of students said they'd feel *comfortable* going to use those services, according to the study published in May 2022. Only 55 percent of men and 47 percent of women agreed that mental health was a priority within their athletic departments.

Marks, the former Washington State receiver, asked me, extremely rhetorically, "[The NCAA] is doing the bare minimum, right?" Another former Division I football player who's candid about his mental health, linebacker Jake Lawler, played at the University of North Carolina at Chapel Hill in the 2018 and 2019 seasons before stepping away from the sport. Lawler went even further than Marks in criticizing the NCAA: "They are a draconian organization with fucking Orwellian policies." He elaborated, describing the NCAA's "for-profit environment." Lawler, though, who dealt with depression and suicidal ideation in college, is quick to give credit to North Carolina's mental health professionals. But he argued that the NCAA's practice of leaving policies up to individual schools isn't right. "The only thing they care about is the spectacle," Lawler said. "And the only way they get the spectacle is through using and abusing the bodies of these [athletes] and not giving them any recourse, not giving them anything else."

In 2017, I wrote an article for *The Ringer* about the gradually increasing but still scarce prevalence of adequate, athlete-specific mental health care on the collegiate level. An online survey with a 36 percent response rate, published in 2017 in *Sports Health*, had shown that just about 39 percent of Division I schools staffed mental health clinicians within their athletic departments or athletic training rooms themselves. That's to say nothing of the much less flush Divisions II and III as well as the National Association of Intercollegiate Athletics (NAIA). "Not every school is Baylor," then WNBA guard DiDi Richards told me in 2022 of her alma mater. "Not every school is [women's basketball powerhouse] UConn." She added that every institution has an obligation to try its best regardless.

In 2022, NAIA schools partnered with Mantra Health, a telehealth provider. The relationship is designed to supplement on-campus mental health care with virtual psychological and psychiatric care for all eligible students (not all people, conditions, and situations lend themselves well to care over a video chat app), but specific attention is being paid to athletes across their campuses. Nora Feldpausch, Mantra's medical director, said this isn't necessarily a matter of an adrift college student finding themselves. It's about making sure they survive their twenties, when the second-leading cause of death is suicide. Mantra seeks out providers trained to deal with athletes in particular. "I think we have to be willing, if we're going to try to create elite athletes, in the same way we don't put crappy shoes on them, we can't give them crappy providers," Feldpausch said.

* * *

Mark Hilinski, whose son Tyler died by suicide in 2018 while studying and playing football at Washington State, said there were 565 athletes attending the school at the time and just one part-time sport psychology specialist, who was not a licensed mental health practitioner. (The school did not respond to a request for confirmation of those numbers.) Back in 2000, Gary Bennett, an associate athletic director and a clinical and sport psychologist who attended the University of Kentucky to play baseball before transferring to Division III Centre College, started part-time at Virginia Tech as a clinical and sport psychologist. (As a student, he was a pitcher until he threw out his arm and got stationed in left field—"where all pitchers go to play," he said.)

Bennett was a trailblazer: He was upped to full-time by 2007, by which point he estimated there were about a total of five full-time positions like his across collegiate athletics. But the landscape changed quickly: By the early 2020s, he said, every Power 5 school had at least one mental health clinician in house—if not two, three, or four.

So why does it matter that schools have dedicated mental health practitioners for the athletic departments specifically? We know they have mental health practitioners available for the general population, yes. But those services are far from perfect, and forcing athletes to leave the safety nets of the athletic department to seek out shared resources elsewhere on campus is not a valid solution for most competitors who feel pressure to keep their emotions bottled up. "The campus counseling center is literally 200 yards away on the other side of the parking lot," Bennett told me for that *Ringer* article. "But it might as well be 200 miles."[2]

For one thing, trying to get an appointment can be extremely difficult. Athletes may have to wait a couple of weeks to even get in for a consultation at the general counseling center, and then they may wait more than a week between appointments. "On top of that, they go into a waiting room with nonathletes. And if they're a higher-profile athlete who's recognizable, before they get out of their appointment, it might be posted on social media that they were in the counseling center," Bennett said.

Josie Nicholson, the assistant athletic director for sport psychology at Ole Miss, also stressed the need of providers to be "culturally competent" in dealing with athletes. "It's its own culture," said the former Loyola New Orleans University soccer player. Not everyone is equipped to understand when students' issues may be tied to their sport and when they may be totally independent of their status as an athlete. Understanding that difference is key to getting an athlete the specialized help they need.

Collegiate athletes also benefit from seeing their mental health practitioners out and about within athletic complexes and having the professionals' work mixed into their normal routines. The then director of behavioral science at Wake Forest Baptist Medical Center, Laura Sudano, along with her colleagues Christopher M. Miles and Greg Collins, did national research published in 2017 that showed that one key to spotting and addressing mental health issues in collegiate athletes is to integrate screenings for mental health care into their physical treatment in the training room. "When you're in the athletic training room, which is oftentimes a place for camaraderie as people are coming in for treatment, it sort of normalizes that experience," Sudano told me for *The Ringer*.[3] (Miles and Sudano are also the authors behind the 2016 survey about mental health professionals in Division I athletic departments.) It also might be easier to open up to a professional when you bump into them at lunchtime, in the weight room, or on the sidelines. "They see us. They get to know us a little bit," Bennett said. "It's not like we're sitting in an office somewhere waiting for people to come see us."

* * *

"Picture the ball going into the hoop. When you're falling asleep, picture that." Those words were more or less the extent of Kate Fagan's interactions with a sport psychology professional at the University of Colorado Boulder in the 2000s. Needless to say, they were not very helpful for her mounting anxiety or even for improving her performance. Even for schools that have the right professionals and more consistent instruction in place, stigma is still in play: "You can have all the resources in the world," Mark Hilinski said. "[Those schools] still have nearly the same problem. . . . We still know there are coaches that just simply don't believe. They don't think mental health is an issue. They think there's tough people and weak people. They're coaching our kids."

The very act of setting foot on campus can be overwhelming for a newly minted college athlete. "When you see yourself as 'I'm a really great basketball player, and I'm gonna be successful,' and all this kind of stuff, and I am the best in my town, and everybody knows me for this, all my accolades and all my praise and all my potential comes from this one thing," Nicholson said. "And now I get on a campus where everybody is as good as I am, and so now I'm no longer The One, and so what is special about me? That deconstructs the sense of self in a way that I think is really difficult to understand." It comes back to that idea of athletic identity foreclosure.

Because of the unnatural fusion between academics and sports that the NCAA necessitates, students have to juggle, well, homework. Bennett described the athletes as having two full-time jobs. "That just is inherently stressful," he said. Although teams can practice only 20 hours a week, that figure doesn't come close to representing how much time students spend on their sports. They might have an hour or two of rehabilitation each day for an injury as well as travel time to and from competition sites. "Pretty soon the number of free hours they have gets whittled down, between going to class, going to study hall, studying, and then the athletics part and trying to get a good night's sleep," Bennett said. "All of a sudden you're down to a handful of hours a day when they're not committed to something."

Athletes who aren't enjoying their sports or are too overwhelmed to continue playing in college might feel stuck. "There's a lot of pressure to continue in the sport even if they don't want to, even if they're out of love with the sport and it's actually a big cause of their mental health suffering," said Reardon, who participated in track and field on the club level in college. "Part of that is a sense of obligation to their family who put a lot of time and resources and maybe money into their success in sport. Maybe they need the scholarship to stay at the university 'cause there's no way their family could afford it otherwise." Even seemingly smaller issues can get to athletes, she said, like how whenever they go home for a break, all anyone asks them about is, say, football. It can then begin to feel like football is their entire identity, and there's no way to quit.

There are also the pressures of social media and, more recently, name, image, and likeness (NIL) to contend with. While social media can be a tool for connection and community as well as raising someone's platform, it has obvious drawbacks, especially for college athletes. You're "able to see how people respond to your performance just by snapping your fingers and turning on your phone," said Kacey Oiness, a part-time counseling and sport psychologist at the University of Nevada, Las Vegas. She was a gymnast at Iowa State University.

Meanwhile, Fagan said, "Is there a positive [to social media]? Sure. Is it a net positive? I don't know about that." It's something she explored in depth in her book *What Made Maddy Run*, about the 2014 suicide of University of Pennsylvania runner Madison Holleran. Fagan chronicles in detail how Holleran's darkness was hidden underneath a well-curated Instagram presence. "Yes, people filter their photos to make them prettier," Fagan wrote in her 2015 ESPN feature that would grow into her book. "People are also often encouraged to put filters on their sadness, to brighten their reality so as not to 'drag down' those around them. The myth still exists that happiness is a choice, which perpetuates the notion of depression as weakness."[4]

Then, closely tied to social media and personal branding, there's NIL. It can be a very good thing in the frustrating world of amateurism: As of July 2021, it allows athletes from across divisions the right to profit off their names, images, and likenesses (read: their identities) via endorsements and publicity. Some prominent football recruits have netted deals in the high six figures or low seven figures, for example. Athletes in other sports cashed in, too. University of Connecticut basketball phenom Paige Bueckers, one of the most well-known athletes in all of college sports at the time NIL entered the game, scored deals with Gatorade, Chegg, StockX, and Crocs.

But while occasionally lucrative, NIL can also put a lot of strain on the thousands of athletes who aren't household names and who still want to get paid (and who deserve to be paid like the workers they are). "Thankfully we're able to profit off that and make money, and that's amazing, but it does add an extra level of stress," Sarah Fuller, the starting goalkeeper for the 2020 Southeastern Conference championship–winning Vanderbilt women's soccer team and later the University of North Texas, told me in 2022 when we talked for *Sports Illustrated*.[5] She also, famously, stepped in as placekicker for a couple of the Vanderbilt football team's games in the fall of 2020. Fuller works with NOCAP Sports as its director of athlete relations. It's a group whose mission is to give all athletes equal access to NIL opportunities. The organization says athletes keep 100 percent of the money they net through deals NOCAP facilitates. (It takes 15 percent from the brand's side.)

Mark Hilinski described the potential athlete thought process surrounding NIL this way: "I thought I was gonna make five grand a month. I'm the backup tackle for pick-a-school, and my parents wanna know why I'm not getting what [starting quarterback] Caleb Williams is getting in Oklahoma." (After my chat with Hilinski, Williams transferred to the University of Southern California.) Although Lawler called NIL "the best thing that's happened to [college] athletes," he added, "if 20 kids are seeing six figures but 65 kids aren't seeing anything, that's not really equitable." So NIL can net athletes a nice influx of cash to spend, save, or send home, but it's not without its own stressors or time commitment in an already packed schedule.

Another relatively new concern for college athletes is the NCAA's online transfer portal database, which allows students who enter it to transfer to other schools. It was built in 2018 to provide more transparency around athletes who wish to change institutions. In several major sports, students can now transfer without sitting out a year, as was previously required.

While the expanded NCAA transfer regulations can be a good thing—some people inevitably need a change—John MacPhee, the CEO of the mental health nonprofit The Jed Foundation, is concerned by the portal's widespread use. In 2020 and 2021, thousands of students tried their luck in it. "They're at a school trying to make connections, trying to get your feet under you, and then because they're not playing as much as they had hoped, they transfer," said MacPhee, himself a former Columbia University basketball center who ended up failing out of school on his first go-round. "Sometimes they're transferring twice. That is setting up all kinds of stressors." MacPhee, whose foundation works primarily with teens and young adults on emotional well-being and suicide prevention, also pointed out that transferring is more likely to be successful for superstars in, say, football, who might be riding the bench at one school and transfer to become the starting quarterback for another team.

Beyond NIL and transfers, there's the ultimate issue: retirement. And make no mistake, retirement does come directly after college for most high-level athletes. Only roughly 2 percent of collegiate athletes go on to play their sport professionally, the NCAA has found. "Everything was so cult in America around college sports," Fagan said. "There wasn't even an opportunity to diversify who I spent time with. I felt like I'd lost not just the sport but a friendship group and the physical presence of the athletic department, where I would spend most of my time. You're losing physical spaces. You're losing friend networks. You're losing the way your body moves in space. It is a whole lot of losses that are happening."

* * *

For all the progress Hainline and others have seen in recent years, fundamental issues remain as college athletes try to navigate their busy, stressful lives. For starters, mental illnesses have not been destigmatized for students (or others) at the same rate. "We're just much more willing to talk about depression and anxiety than we are to talk about some of the other issues," Hainline said. He gave PTSD as an example, citing that 36 percent of female athletes had experienced sexual violence in college, according to a 2022 *Journal of Interpersonal Violence* study. "I don't think we've made great headway there," Hainline said. "We're certainly talking about it and investigating it."

I talked to MacPhee, the JED CEO, in September 2022. He said that even over the previous year, the ways people have spoken about collegiate athlete mental health have changed. There are athletes with severe mental illnesses, like Hainline mentioned above, and then there are those who develop anxiety and related symptoms due to the current climate, featuring a loss of reproductive rights with the overturning of *Roe v. Wade*, police violence, anti-Asian hate, and more. "The answer is not do a mindfulness app, spend more time outside, talk to a therapist online, draw in an adult coloring book, and you'll be able to cope better with all this stuff going on," MacPhee said. He said the students he speaks with—athletes and not—are agitated. They rightly see what's happening in the world as an emergency as opposed to a personal mental health crisis.

One other area where there's obvious room for growth is equipping Division II and III schools with the appropriate resources. At one point recently, Connole said, athletes at the Division I level were almost three times as likely to have mental health and mental performance services available to them. On the conference level, momentum is building. In the fall of 2021, the Big Ten, Pac-12, and Atlantic Coast Conference formed an alliance to address mental health issues among athletes called Teammates for Mental Health. Collectively, they represent more than 27,000 college athletes. But the news seemed to be focused mostly on awareness as opposed to requiring or even recommending more resources. (Each of the three conferences also has its own mental health working group, initiative, or cabinet, all created in the 2010s.)

Hainline points to the Mid-American Conference (MAC) as a pioneer when it comes to athlete mental health care within the NCAA. Commissioner Jon Steinbrecher, who took up his post in 2009, had quite a similar experience to Hainline's. Steinbrecher acknowledged to me that mental health wasn't on his radar when he started his new role; rather, it was students who pushed the issue. In the 2014–2015 school year, Steinbrecher remembered, he asked students which areas the conference could afford to work on. (Every year or two, Steinbrecher said, he takes a tour of athlete-led advisory committees at every MAC school.) The students told him: mental health.

So Steinbrecher assembled an athlete well-being task force to spend about 18 months digging into questions about how the MAC could bolster its support of its students' mental health. Education turned out to be a big area for improvement, so students began spreading the "it's okay to not be okay" message in the hopes of eliminating stigma. The conference has also hosted a Taking MACtion Summit every year since 2016. It's half dedicated to discussing mental health and half dedicated to discussing diversity and inclusion (a sprawling issue that itself greatly correlates to mental health outcomes for athletes). But MAC member schools have upped the numbers of mental health professionals available on campuses in recent years, Steinbrecher said, adding that the conference was early enough to the awareness campaign idea that back then he had a "drum beating" of people from across the NCAA reaching out to ask about how to replicate its success.

If this all sounds to you like the MAC might have a nice awareness campaign going but not much else, know I had the same thought. I challenged Steinbrecher on this point and urged him to share what (m)action he's taken that goes beyond awareness. "I'm a little bit separated from that since I'm here [in my office] and not on campus," he acknowledged. Then he made a good point: With a rotating cast of college students, coaches, and administrators, in a way, you're starting from square one every semester with a new crop of faces and new relationships. Steinbrecher added, "This isn't just a switch you flip and you're off and running." So those awareness campaigns, repetitive and shallow as they might seem to an outsider like me who hears about scores of them, are important to frequently spearhead on campuses.

***

Suicides in the NCAA offer a glaring reminder of how much progress is still to be made on caring for mentally ill athletes. "I think there have been some major catastrophic cases in college athletics—student-athlete suicides—that have really raised the alarm from a crisis management standpoint," Connole said. Tyler Hilinski's death was perhaps the highest-profile college athlete suicide in recent memory. "Unfortunately, football's always gonna be the [sport] that gets people's attention, and then his position, [plus coach] Mike Leach being well known," said Nicholson, who hosts the *UNIT3D* podcast for Hilinski's Hope Foundation.

Hilinski's parents, Mark and Kym, realize the role their family tragedy has played in the larger conversation around mental health care for athletes. "It took so many other student-athletes sharing their story and struggling, and sadly some of them passed as well," Kym said. Today, she and Mark advocate tirelessly, traveling to schools to talk to students and staff about the lessons from Tyler's death that may be able to help save others' lives.

Marks graduated from Washington State a couple of years before Hilinski died. But their relationship goes way back, having known each other since they were about 11 years old. Marks used to work out with Kelly Hilinski, Tyler's older brother. "Everything was pointing to him going to be a starter next year," Marks said of Tyler. "He finally got a shot, and we were all very excited for him. And then you get the news, it was just very shocking, and it made us all look at our own experiences. Are we okay? Are the boys all right?"

A few years before Hilinski's death, there was Holleran's. She died by suicide at age 19 in 2014, during her second semester of school. Due in part to Fagan's writing about Holleran, first for ESPN in 2015 and later in her book, the death commanded national attention, just like Hilinski's would years later.

"I do think there's something about our society's need to understand, 'Oh, that's how bad it is,'" Fagan said. "Because otherwise, how do you explain to people? We have this need for these full story arcs that make sense in our mind. Even though we can't say A led to B led to C led to D, we know the outcome of D is so incredibly tragic that we are compelled to understand all of the steps along the way, even if we're not sure they all add up to something." Each suicide serves as a grim reminder of the country's mental health crisis—one that certainly reaches far beyond college sports to touch every corner of our lives. But it's often their suffering that catches our eyes.

The tragedies kept coming during COVID-19. As everyone's well-being worsened in the pandemic—Nicholson called it a "mental health shitshow"—college athletes were no exception. Added Hainline, "There was such uncertainty. The athletes are so used to their goal-setting behaviors, and they have a sense of control, and they know how to fall down and pick themselves up. Well, everything was just taken away from them." Rates of mental exhaustion, anxiety, and depression were one and a half to two times higher among NCAA athletes during the pandemic than they were beforehand, the governing body's survey showed.

A full two years into the pandemic, the spring of 2022 seemed particularly fraught for college athletes. At least five died by suicide between that March and May—four of them women. The first was Katie Meyer, a 22-year-old goalkeeper and captain of Stanford's women's soccer team who had helped her team to a national championship in 2019. She rose to prominence after making a pair of crucial saves in the penalty kick shoot-out against the University of North Carolina. Gina and Steve Meyer had spoken with their daughter just hours before her death. "She was excited," Gina told *Today* just days after Katie's suicide. "She had a lot on her plate. She had a lot going on. But she was happy. She was in great spirits."[6]

Katie Meyer wasn't the only championship-caliber athlete lost to suicide in the spring of 2022. Lauren Bernett died about a month and a half later. She was the James Madison University softball team's starting catcher and had played with the team in its Women's College World Series–winning campaign in her last full season. The day before her death, she was named the Colonial Athletic Association's Player of the Week. The final at bat of her final season resulted in a home run. "Really sad," Oklahoma State University softball coach Kenny Gajewski said following Bernett's suicide, as tears welled up. "It's sad because it's become quite normal."[7]

Between the deaths of Meyer and Bernett, there were the suicides of Wisconsin runner Sarah Shulze, Northern Michigan runner Jayden Hill, and Binghamton lacrosse player Robert Martin. And those are just the ones we know about from that spring, the ones that made headlines.

Courtney Coppersmith recognized that she could've been one of those athletes. I spoke to the PhD student at the University of Maryland, Baltimore County, in 2022, about half a year after that wave of Division I suicides. Years earlier, the softball pitcher quietly struggled as a freshman. She wouldn't wear a seat belt when driving and went on late-night runs despite her campus not having a blue-light security system at the time. Coppersmith didn't actively try to harm herself, but she wouldn't have cared had something happened to her, either. "Whatever happens, happens," she recalled thinking.

Coppersmith was also barely sleeping. "It would be points where it'd be okay, it was 3 o'clock in the morning on days we'd have to be out at 5:30, and I'm still awake," she said. "Or if we had an off day or something I'd be like, oh well, lying in bed, *why go to class?* I'm a big school person, so that wasn't good."

She eventually came forward in an essay she wrote for an organization called Reviving Baseball in Inner Cities. Every player on every team entered in the tournament had to write an essay for a contest judged by Jackie Robinson's daughter, Sharon, about how the player's values relate to the baseball legend's. Coppersmith, who played for Harrisburg, was shocked to learn she won the contest for writing about her struggle with depression and anxiety. Having her mental illness out in the open let others, like friends and athletic trainers, support her. And when Coppersmith did get into a car accident in December 2019, while she wasn't wearing a seat belt, she found herself glad to be alive afterward.

"If I would've continued to stay in that mindset and [my story] wouldn't have come out, I think it could've potentially gone that way [of suicide]," Coppersmith said. "I can't guarantee, but it's like [*shrugs*], most people didn't know that that was what was going to happen with any of them either."

* * *

Much of the recent change, especially in terms of amping up the volume on the existing mental health dialogue on college campuses, has been at the grassroots level: More athletes have been speaking out about what they've been through—and asking for the resources they need. "Gen Z is not hesitant to speak truth to power," Dartmouth's Connole said.

Once some athletes started speaking up on both the collegiate and the professional level, others followed suit. "There was a stigma that was pretty considerable with that, but that has been shifting, and I think in large part because so many athletes in a courageous way have been telling their story," said the NCAA's Hainline. Lawler, the former University of North Carolina football player, became one of five founders of UNCUT Chapel Hill, a nonprofit that strives to tell the school's athletes' stories in their own words, often relating to their mental health. UNCUT came together in fall 2018, formally launching its multimedia content the following year.

But Lawler's personal journey to UNCUT was a long one. He had endured depression since age 12 or 13. "We do such a terrible, awful job of teaching mental health," he said. "Kids like me, for example, will be depressed for years and not know what it is." He didn't love playing football. Rather, he played in an (unsuccessful) effort to stop the bullying he was facing. He also played to lessen his parents' financial burden.

Lawler's first suicide attempt came in 2015. The thought of his family stopped him. "I just bottled all of it up, and I just focused on school and focused on being the best student, being the son, being the best football player, being the best teammate I could be but never really focused on being the best person," he said. When he went to make his second suicide attempt, when he was in college, he couldn't even say why he didn't go through with it. "Honestly, it was one of those situations like, if the wind blew a little bit harder. . . . There wasn't necessarily a reason why I didn't [kill myself]."

With the help of his roommate, Lawler started opening up to more people: his coach, his teammates, his family. UNCUT also played a huge role. He started chatting with fellow Black athletes about what it was like attending a primarily white institution. He found strength in vulnerability and also strength in writing and talking out his own story through UNCUT and his personal blog.

Meanwhile, students across campuses were having similar reckonings—both personal and global—about what it means to be collegiate athletes and grapple with the mental illness of themselves or their friends. In November 2017, Taylor Ricci and Nathan Braaten started the nonprofit Dam Worth It at Oregon State University. The gymnast and the soccer player, respectively, got to know each other after each had lost a teammate to suicide in the preceding year. They spent five hours at a coffee shop plotting what they could do about the mental health crisis within campus athletics and came up with Dam Worth It.

Similar to UNCUT, which itself has spread to multiple college campuses, Dam Worth It focuses on storytelling and raising awareness of stigma. It also was awarded $60,000 from the Pac-12 to survey hundreds of collegiate athletes across the conference in the 2018–2019 academic year and get a better sense of what that population is up against. Ricci believes that at the time, the 638 athletes and 400 staff members who responded made up the largest mental health survey ever done in the conference. Eighty-five percent of the athletes surveyed reported that their stress levels were at a 5 out of 10 or above. Nearly one-quarter of respondents had been diagnosed with a mental health disorder. More than 80 percent of those surveyed across 11 institutions wanted to see more mental health resources on their campuses.

"At the time when Nathan and I were students at Oregon State, there was not a full-time counselor for student-athletes," said Ricci, who has experienced both anxiety and depression, though she was never formally diagnosed with either. "We were going through the counseling and psychological services on campus. I reached out to them, and it took me a couple of weeks to get my first appointment. By the time I sat down on my couch at my first appointment, I was like, 'I don't really want to talk about this anymore.'"

Dam Worth It Company has spread to at least a handful of branches at other schools (including a high school). Its stated mission is to "be the gold standard in higher education for establishing, implementing, and sustaining peer-led mental health awareness campaigns."[8] The subtext, arguably, is that there's a great need for peer-led mental health awareness campaigns because institutions themselves aren't adequately filling in their gaps in coverage and in some cases are actively staying silent on mental health. Ricci said the NCAA and its member schools are doing better now than they were when she was in school less than a decade ago but that there's still plenty of room for growth. "Now there's definitely a good lens and a good frame that the NCAA is placing on mental health and prioritizing for student-athletes, but the answer is going to be there can always be more," she said. "Schools can always do more. Coaches can always do more."

Of course, these student-driven campaigns could go even further. Beyond awareness through (still helpful) measures like handing out shirts at football games, they could directly pressure their schools' administrators to take specific actions, like employing more mental health professionals within athletic departments. They could also support efforts to unionize NCAA athletes, which, if successful, would surely guarantee employees (the athletes) more comprehensive mental health care (and, you know, other handy resources designed to promote mental health, like wages).

* * *

PART III

THE DIAGNOSIS

Coping with What You've Got

CHAPTER 8

Substance Use

From Alcohol and Cannabis to Psychedelics

DANIEL CARCILLO STARTED PLAYING HOCKEY AT AGE FOUR, WHICH meant he started hitting—and getting hit—at age four. The sport was an emotional release for him. His path to the NHL was bumpy, though. Carcillo, from Ontario, played as a teenager in the Canadian Hockey League (CHL), a system of three junior leagues that funnel athletes to the NHL. He was 17 during the Sarnia Sting's 2002–2003 season, and he had no idea how hockey was about to continue shaping him. Carcillo and 11 other rookies that year, he said, survived hazing, bullying, verbal and sexual harassment, and physical and sexual assault.

"Hockey's very cult-like, where you get hazing and a lot of really gnarly stuff," he told me nearly two decades later for *Sports Illustrated*.[1] Already an angry kid, he became even more so because of the abuse he described suffering. In 2020, Carcillo and another former CHL player, Garrett Taylor, filed a class-action lawsuit against the system and its member leagues outlining a host of specific allegations. Among them, per the lawsuit, were that players were forced to masturbate in front of teammates and coaches; consume saliva, urine, semen, and feces; and engage with animals in a sexual manner. They also had hockey sticks, brooms, and food forced into their anuses, Carcillo and Taylor said in the lawsuit.

"I fought 164 times in the NHL," said Carcillo, a winger nicknamed "Car Bomb" who had a nine-year pro career. "[The abuse] really formed me into that type of person." For the first half of his time in the NHL, Carcillo said he didn't want to think about the physical and emotional pain he was in. At one point, he said, when he was 23, his team had him undergo two surgeries in 10 days: a stapling of his abdomen to his pelvis and an arthroscopic hip procedure. In the aftermath, he said, he was prescribed strong painkillers without being educated about their addictive properties. "I was like, 'Woah, what is this?'" Carcillo said. "I had a lot of emotional trauma, physical trauma, and it just took everything away."

So Carcillo took painkillers, and he also drank a lot of alcohol. After the adrenaline rush of playing in a game, he'd drink and take a sleep aid to come down. His performance suffered, and so did his mental health. That was all while he kept racking up concussions—he'd end his career with seven. (Carcillo was one of more than 100 former NHL players who joined a 2016 lawsuit against the league, alleging that it did not do enough to prevent trauma or warn athletes of the risks of violent play. The suit was settled two years later, without the NHL admitting any liability.)

During Carcillo's career, two years after his introduction to painkillers, he sought out help for his addiction and ended up in rehab at The Canyon in Malibu, California. There, in addition to getting sober, he learned about meditation and breathing exercises. "I started living the right way," he said. And his performance improved as a result. In each of his last four years in the league, his teams went to the Stanley Cup final. He won the Cup twice. The only problem? He still didn't feel well.

To make matters worse, Steve Montador, a close friend and fellow NHL player who helped Carcillo through his substance use issues, died in February 2015, less than a year after retiring. He was 35 and later found to have CTE, a brain condition diagnosed posthumously and thought to be caused by concussions and repeated hits to the head. Montador's official cause of death was listed as accidental overdose. Just a month later, Carcillo notched his seventh concussion. "I was isolating," Carcillo said. "I wanted nothing to do with my [young] kid. I didn't want to go to the rink."

The year that Montador died, Carcillo was experiencing a slew of symptoms that his seventh concussion only worsened: When we spoke, he quickly rattled off light sensitivity, slurred speech, headaches, head pressure, migraines, impulse control issues, insomnia, anxiety, depression, and suicidal ideation. His team, the Chicago Blackhawks, had won the Stanley Cup after the 2014–2015 season, and Carcillo couldn't even bring himself to attend the banner raising.

Montador's death and Carcillo's retirement launched what he calls his "brain health journey." He went to brain banks to research CTE and read up on scientific papers. He started seeing neurologists and testing out different modalities: acupuncture, hyperbaric chambers, you name it. Carcillo said that over five years, he spent $400,000 and still wasn't feeling any better. With three kids under age seven, he started planning for suicide. He felt ashamed of his impulse-control issues and how often he was fighting with his wife.

But everything changed for him in 2019, when a former teammate (whom Carcillo declined to name) reached out. "Come to this farm, man," he urged. It was ostensibly a trip to learn about cannabis and CBD. Carcillo needed a break to reset himself, so he said yes. Once there, the friend and a biochemist surprised him with a large dose of psilocybin, commonly known as magic mushrooms. We'll get more into what happened next and what Carcillo is up to now, but he illustrates an important concept: Athletes—current and former—take substances in a variety of ways, either to the detriment of their health or as a boon to it, when used carefully.

* * *

The culture of alcohol and drugs is pervasive throughout society, and sports are no different. Royce White, the basketball player who challenged the NBA to offer better mental health care for athletes, explained as much to me for *The Ringer* in 2018. He pointed to the NBA's partnership with Anheuser-Busch as fostering an unhealthy environment at basketball games. (He also argued that mental illness had been an issue in leagues like the NBA for decades, with many players using cocaine in the 1970s and 1980s.)

Lee Dorpfeld, the director of sport psychology at the University of South Florida, Tampa, has a subspecialty in substance abuse and, like

White, points toward our culture at sporting events as part of the problem. "Human beings like to find ways to not feel certain emotions and feelings when they don't have to. And it's socially acceptable, promoted. Some of your biggest sponsors in sports and entertainment are alcohol companies," he said. "The idea of the fan going to a game and having a beer or whatever in the crowd is a common societal norm for attending sporting events."

In general, athletes—necessarily very particular about what they put in their bodies—use substances less than the general population, said Claudia Reardon, a professor and psychiatrist who works with athletes at the University of Wisconsin. But there are important exceptions. Take alcohol, for example. Athletes are thought to consume less than nonathletes, but they engage in higher rates of binge drinking (typically defined as five or more drinks for a man and four or more for a woman), especially during their offseasons. "There can be a sense of, during the season I'm extremely rigid and do all the things that are helpful and positive for my body and then, gosh, I earned it to party a little bit in the offseason," she said. "That can get to dangerous degrees and then [continue] sometimes even within the season for purposes of celebrating wins or consoling losses."

That's a phenomenon that Erin Rubenking, University of Colorado Boulder's associate director of psychological health and performance, has also observed. "It is that go hard or go home mentality of *okay, if we're going to go out, we're going to do it right*," she said. Rubenking also explained that, as a casual athlete herself (a trail runner), she sees a lot of similarities between athletes and people with addictions. "There is such a focus and dedication, and it's like, all or nothing," she added.

While the primary reason athletes use substances is social, in many cases, they are self-medicating, Dorpfeld said. Anecdotally, he explained, he can often tell what comorbid mental illness an athlete might be struggling with based on which drugs they turn to for coping. "Somebody with anxiety is probably not going to want to use cocaine or some amphetamine. It's going to speed them up and make them more anxious," he said. "They're going to want to take something that calms them down. Somebody who's depressed is probably not going to want something that makes them feel depressed. They're going to want something that lifts them up." Emet Marwell, who briefly played field hockey at Mount Holyoke and is bipolar, said he's still working on his relationship to alcohol. "[Substance use is] definitely an accessible coping mechanism," he said. "Way more accessible than therapy or meds."

The most common substances that athletes use, much like the general population, are alcohol and cannabis. But professionals like Dorpfeld also see athletes who are addicted to painkillers, crack or cocaine, and benzodiazepines (depressants commonly used to treat anxiety). Soccer icon and former U.S. women's national team goalkeeper Briana Scurry, part of the famed 1999 World Cup–winning squad, wrote about self-medicating in her 2022 book with Wayne Coffey, *My Greatest Save*. She detailed the long road to recovery after sustaining a debilitating head injury in the game a decade earlier. "I prided myself on being strong and self-reliant, and now I was as far from that as you can get, desperate and vulnerable," she wrote. "I said nothing and suffered in silence, mostly gutting through it, sometimes self-medicating with Vicodin and alcohol, trying to get my brain back and taking the edge off the jackhammer headaches that pounded on me all day long."[2]

Athletes are about as likely to use substances on the college level as in the pros, Dorpfeld said. On the pro level, though, the substances of choice may differ because, he explained, "their body is their profession. . . . Nutrition, sleep, supplementation, all the things that they do. Putting excessive chemicals or putting large amounts of alcohol or other substances actually gets in the way of them being able to perform, which is what they're getting paid to do."

There's also the matter of the college setting normalizing alcohol and cannabis consumption. "[Binge drinking] seems normal to them," Rubenking said. About 42 percent of college athletes reported having engaged in binge drinking, according to the NCAA's 2017 substance use survey of about 23,000 athletes. Meanwhile, about a quarter of college athletes use cannabis, according to the same survey. In 2022, the NCAA raised its threshold for a positive THC test from 35 nanograms per milliliter to 150, which lines up with the threshold of the World Anti-Doping Agency (WADA), the entity that governs drug use across Olympic sports. College sports' governing body also minimized penalties for first, second, and third infractions, dictating that as long as athletes who test positive comply with their school's education plan requirements, they won't lose eligibility for any of their regular-season contests.

Cannabis could be a safer alternative to opiates for pain management, said Dorpfeld, who made clear to me that he's not advocating for *any* substance use, just that he's coming at it from a place of curiosity and minimizing harm if possible. "There's a lot of pain and a lot of stuff that comes from chronically beating the hell out of your body for years," he said. "So if we can find a way to help people that have chronic pain as a result of multiple years of participating in high levels of athletics— without them getting hooked on something or becoming dependent on it biologically—then why aren't we looking into that as an alternative?"

Cannabis, of course, is a hotly debated, highly politicized drug, including within sports. Sha'Carri Richardson brought the long-simmering issue to the forefront in track the year before. Days after the emerging star won the 100 meters at the U.S. Olympic trials in 2021 in Eugene, Oregon, her drug test results came back positive for cannabis, a WADA-banned substance.

Richardson used cannabis, which is fully legal in Oregon, after learning via a reporter that her biological mother had died, she told NBC shortly after her test results came back. "[I'm] not making an excuse or looking for any empathy in my case, but, however, being in that position in my life, finding out something like that, something that I would say is probably one of the biggest things that have impacted me . . . that definitely was a very heavy topic on me," she said. "People don't understand what it's like to have to . . . go in front of the world and put on a face and hide my pain. Who am I to tell you how to cope when you're dealing with the pain or you're dealing with a struggle that you haven't experienced before or that you thought you never would have to deal with?"[3]

LaTisha Bader, the chief clinical officer for Denver Women's Recovery, a gender-specific intensive outpatient program, specializes in substance use and addiction. "What integrity for [Richardson]," she said. "I am ever so impressed with her." Bader, like other experts, believes that cannabis is not helpful to athletes' performances. Even so, it remains on WADA's and the NCAA's banned lists as if it *could* engineer better performance. In recent years, leagues including the NFL and NBA have downgraded or stopped testing for cannabis. "I have never seen a substance change—transform—in such a short time [during my career]," Bader said. "Alcohol's been alcohol. . . . Cocaine has been cocaine." She means both the substance itself and the conversation surrounding it.

The case for athletes' cannabis use isn't quite so simple, though, as Bader and others realize. "We are seeing concerning things, especially with the potency levels now," Rubenking said. "Just the age range that I'm working with, 18 to 22, you're at higher risk for some of these negative side effects of cannabis use." Often, even though it's legal in certain states and not necessarily correlated with using hard drugs, using cannabis can harm athletes' performance and mental health—even as they think it's helping. Athletes whom Rubenking works with—and she sees about 200 athletes of the school's 300-plus in an individual or group setting every semester—tend to tell her cannabis is calming and helpful for dealing with stress. But over the long term, Rubenking sees the *opposite* in those who use regularly, perhaps a couple of times a week or more, especially at a high potency. "We see increases in anxiety," she said. "We see increases in depression."

David R. McDuff, a clinical professor of psychiatry at the University of Maryland School of Medicine who has long worked with athletes, has seen cannabis transform as well—and not necessarily for the better—when it comes to athlete use during his long career. "I worked at a large university from 1997 to 2009, and then I left and went back again 10 years later, and the landscape had changed so substantially with respect to cannabis use," he said. "Far more athletes were using cannabis, and far more athletes were using cannabis daily. Of those who were using daily, invariably their grades started to fall. They ended up on academic probation. Their commitment to their lifting programs, nutrition, their sport in practice, began to decline. Their general motivation tended to drop." So while we praise athletes like Richardson for their courage in speaking out about their mental health, the larger question of cannabis's role in sport—if it should have any at all—is tricky.

***

In some cases, alcohol can be even trickier to address in elite athletes—it's fully legal and not thought to be performance enhancing, so athletes aren't drug tested for it. The ubiquity can also make it harder for athletes to realize they need to seek help. Riley Sheahan, a former NHL center who as of late 2022 was playing professionally in Switzerland, told me his use of alcohol felt pretty standard to him at the time. "Yeah, I definitely was abusing it, but not to a point that was totally different than what other people were around my age and my group of friends [were doing]," he said. "I just find it's such a normalcy now for athletes—for anybody—who's growing up and experiencing a social life. It's such a normal thing to go out and overdrink and abuse yourself that way."

In 2012, two years after Sheahan was drafted, he was stopped in his car in Michigan wearing a purple *Teletubbies* costume with a blood-alcohol level of 0.30, more than four times the legal limit. He was also underage and carrying a teammate's ID. It was his second arrest on alcohol-related charges. "I had people making a joke out of it when it was something that was hard to deal with," he said. After pleading guilty, Sheahan was sentenced to one year of probation, a $1,325 fine, 49 hours on a work crew, and a victim impact class.

Around the same time, in Sheahan's first couple of years as a professional, a prospect in the Detroit Red Wings' organization, he also started feeling the weight of anxiety and depression. After the DUI, he got started on psychiatric medicine and, he said, dug himself out of a hole. Sheahan considers coping an "ongoing process." In 2021, he started hosting a podcast called *Speak Your Mind*, where he chats with fellow athletes about mental health.

When athletes in particular have substance use disorders, there's a huge stigma associated with them. "Some coaches will just essentially unplug from that athlete and go work with others who haven't developed serious problems with substances," said McDuff. Swimming great Michael Phelps had long struggled without seeking help—there was his first DUI, in 2004, and then a controversy and subsequent USA Swimming suspension over his being photographed with a bong—but, similar to Sheahan, he eventually reached a tipping point. That was his second DUI, in 2014. "I feel like at that point of not wanting to be alive for those 24, 48 hours, that was the kind of thing where I was like, *All right, am I just going to give up?*" he told me for *Sports Illustrated* in 2022. "*Or am I going to find a different road, a different answer?*"[4] Despite the stigma, he decided to go to rehab.

CC Sabathia, a retired superstar pitcher for Cleveland's baseball team (now the Guardians) and then the New York Yankees, also decided to go to rehab for alcohol use, just a year after Phelps, in 2015. His road there, like Phelps's, was long and winding. Drafted out of high school in 1998, Sabathia spent offseasons for much of his career drinking. A lot. "I would routinely drink until I blacked out," he wrote with Chris Smith in his excellent 2021 memoir, *Till the End*. "Unconsciousness was actually the preferred outcome, because I was not a happy drunk—most nights if I got loaded and didn't just pass out, I'd want to fight someone. Anyone."[5]

During seasons, he showed a little bit of restraint, or so he thought. He would drink on his off days but dry out two days before a start. After the game, he'd head to the shower with a tall Gatorade cup and refill it on his way home to Jersey. Sabathia said he wasn't totally out of place in doing so. "It was the culture of our clubhouse at the time; I certainly wasn't the only one leaving the ballpark carrying a giant Gatorade cup cocktail," he wrote. "But I was the only one who would keep drinking hard for the next three days, sweating some of the booze out during a workout in the afternoon and then drinking until I passed out at night."[6]

Sabathia knew that his drinking was problematic, but, as he wrote, "recognizing a pattern is one thing; wanting to change it is something else."[7] He thought he wasn't an alcoholic because he didn't drink every day and could go weeks without it if he wanted to. Eventually, Sabathia wrote, he was tired of hiding. So he told team officials ahead of the 2015 playoffs that he was going to rehab—he knew his issue couldn't wait any longer. But, in his own words, he showed up to the rehab facility, Silver Hill in Connecticut, "hammered."[8]

Once an elite athlete makes the sometimes difficult decision to go to rehab, there's the matter of sorting out the logistics: It's tough for anyone to take a break from their life to address substance use, but for athletes, it might mean stepping away from their sport, livelihood, and main source of joy and stress relief. McDuff said even intensive outpatient treatment (meaning someone does not stay over in the hospital each night) typically occurs during the daytime or early evening, interfering with training. "If they're out of season, it might work, but there's really no out of season," McDuff said, acknowledging the reality that athletes' schedules are booked up year-round. A football player likely has a spring season to train during, for example, and similar offseason work is required in many other sports.

Athletes might also worry about how sobering up will affect their performance. "What if I needed to drink to pitch well?" Sabathia asked himself. "Maybe that doesn't sound completely logical, but in my first few days at rehab, that's how I was thinking."[9] But eventually, he bought into treatment, telling Robin Roberts of *Good Morning America* in his first interview after the program ended, "There was no other option for me but to get help."[10]

While in rehab, Sabathia was inspired by the 1981 book *Five O'Clock Comes Early* by Bob Welch with journalist George Vecsey. It was, like Sabathia's own book would become three decades later, an essential chronicle of life in professional baseball dealing with and recovering from alcoholism. Welch was a pitcher for the Los Angeles Dodgers when he went to rehab at The Meadows in 1980, just two years into his time in the majors. Vecsey, in his prologue to the book, noted, "This was an unusual step in 1980; people did not talk about treatment back then."[11] It was quite the understatement.

One thing Welch, who died at age 57 in 2014 after breaking his neck in an accidental fall in his bathroom, made perfectly clear was that baseball wasn't to blame for his alcoholism, but it did make using awfully convenient for him. "There's beer just for snapping your fingers in the clubhouse, there're all kinds of parties, and you're on the road a hundred nights a year," Welch wrote. "You walk through a hotel lobby, and people are standing in line to buy you a drink. It's easy to say yes, if you're inclined to say yes in the first place."[12]

Unlike with Sabathia, going to rehab was not exactly Welch's choice. His alcoholism was not hidden very well from the team, which arranged for his treatment and covered his time at The Meadows with insurance. Not every athlete is so privileged, but Welch set an example for Sabathia and others who would follow. In fact, Sabathia wrote, "Once I returned to the game, at least once a month a player from another team would come up to me on the field asking about rehab: 'What's it like? How did you do it? How did you know you needed to go?' They weren't just asking because they were curious; they were struggling, too."[13]

The team environment and close camaraderie among athletes may be something that they and those who treat them can harness to strengthen recovery systems, Dorpfeld said. "What happens when you have multiple athletes on a team who are trying to impact their behavior, change their behavior?" he asked. "Can you get them to work together and help each other because the concept of a team is incredibly familiar to them?"

* * *

Until now, we've considered mostly substances that have the potential to harm athletes. But a growing number of people, including athletes and former athletes, believe that *when used properly*, certain drugs—psychedelics in particular—can actually improve their mental health in the long term. So let's get back to Daniel Carcillo and the psilocybin he was surprised with on the farm (in a city he declined to name, where the drugs are decriminalized). What might it be like to have a healthier relationship with substances? He was close to finding out.

Carcillo told me those first couple of hours after taking the psilocybin were the worst he'd ever experienced. But, he added, "I was ready to take my own life. I was willing to try anything." He was purging and dry heaving, walking around in a circle on the farm. His friend and a guide got him to relax a bit. Once the purging stopped, he lay down on a couch. "I remember looking at my friend and this guide after I started to feel pretty good, and they came to me as saints," Carcillo said. "I remember one of them saying, 'Hey, man, this is what we wanted to show you. We want you on our team [figuratively].' I'll never forget: 'You want me? I'm such a loser. Why do you want me on your team?' 'No, man, you're not.'"

At the time, Carcillo didn't understand the magnitude of the ceremony—what many call their experiences with psilocybin and other psychedelics. How could you, when you're busy purging? But as he went home and resumed his life (with a microdosing regimen in hand), he noticed his negative self-talk turning to positive self-talk. Slowly, he felt better. His symptoms faded, and he said brain scans and blood tests at the six-month mark and beyond proved he had changed for the better. At the same time, Carcillo's careful to mention that, just like any other psychiatric medication, no psychedelic is a miracle drug. "Psilocybin's a tool," he said. "If I didn't wake up this morning and work out and hydrate and get eight hours of sleep last night, nothing's going to work for me. And nothing will work for others. I truly believe that."

* * *

Daniel Poneman, an NBA agent who has used psychedelics himself, said he understands why some athletes and former athletes are drawn to them over traditional psychiatric medications. "Professional athletes are seen to so many like superheroes," he told me for *Sports Illustrated* in 2022. "And superheroes don't want to seem flawed. They don't want to seem wounded. They don't want to seem vulnerable. And to take an SSRI [selective serotonin reuptake inhibitor] is to admit that you have depression."[14]

So are the benefits Carcillo said he experienced replicable? Are psychedelics like psilocybin a salve for mental illness and traumatic brain injuries? Courtney Campbell Walton is a postdoctoral research fellow at the University of Melbourne who had published, along with Monash University psychedelic researcher Paul Liknaitzky, possibly the only paper on psychedelics in elite sport at the time we spoke. He said in 2022, "There's this interesting back-and-forth that I see in psychedelic research, of one group describing these as gonna change the world and change psychiatry forever, and one group that's like, 'They don't work, and it's all a scam.'"[15]

The classic psychedelics are considered psilocybin, LSD (acid), mescaline (in peyote), and DMT (in ayahuasca). Lethal overdose, for most people, is not a concern, said psychologist Matthew W. Johnson, a professor of psychiatry and behavioral science at the Johns Hopkins School of Medicine, one of the leading institutions for psychedelics research. MDMA (ecstasy), PCP, ketamine, toad, and salvia also belong to the psychedelics class. Walton and other experts echoed Poneman's earlier point to me, that there's a certain appeal to these medicines over traditional psychiatric drugs because they're a "shiny, exciting new thing," Walton said.

Anna Symonds, a professional rugby player in the United States who retired in 2021 and took various psychedelics during her career, said traditional antidepressants, in her case SSRIs, had not worked for her. "They made me feel much worse," she said. "And there were all these weird side effects." Among them, she said, was the fact that she became suicidal while taking them. (Antidepressants and all traditional psychiatric medicines come with a lot of complications and side effects, but they also do help a lot of people, self included.)

Antidepressants didn't work for Rashad Evans, either. He is a former Ultimate Fighting Championship (UFC) light heavyweight champion who retired in 2018. When he tore his anterior cruciate ligament beforehand and ended up unable to compete on and off for the better part of two years, the weight of his divorce hit him, and he fell into a depression. "It was difficult because at the time I was so into my career, so into my sport, that I just had tunnel vision on all that was happening on the inside," Evans said. "I just poured all the hurt, all the frustration into competing. But then when I didn't have it anymore, all those things came to the surface and I really started to get a true glimpse of the collateral damage that had happened."

He felt empty and traumatized by the life experiences he had been setting aside so he could maintain the image of a stereotypical alpha male fighter. "I climbed to the top of my sport, but I still wasn't satisfied," he said. "I've rubbed shoulders with people who you'd call the biggest stars in the world. . . . I've had my chance to do some amazing things and see some amazing things, go to some amazing places. But none of it was satisfying. It just didn't fill me up."

Trying traditional psychiatric medicine was "the worst feeling ever," he said, and his suicidal thoughts increased. With psychedelics, on the other hand, he felt more clearheaded, more in touch with both himself and others around him. Evans, like Carcillo, stopped feeling the need to drink alcohol. In fact, when Evans tried drinking, he threw up.

Symonds described her use of psychedelics as offering relief to childhood and adulthood trauma she had bottled up. "It seemed to, for me, really accelerate processing some of those things in an overarching way," she said. "It was almost like it helped swallow them whole, break them into smaller pieces, and maybe spit them back a little less toxic."

Certainly not everyone is attracted to psychedelics on that basis of avoiding traditional psychiatric medicine—they're just looking for the best answers they can find, in whatever form they might take. "I've seen all kinds of patients in these various studies, and some people have no aversion at all," Johnson said. "They're all for plain old standard Western medicine, but they've tried it all, and they just want something that works. Nothing's worked yet. So part of it's that. 'My god, I'd love it if Prozac had worked for me.'"

Every reputable expert will acknowledge that there's much more research to be done before they can definitively say that psychedelics are helpful for mental health purposes, but there's reason for excitement based on early returns for psilocybin and other medications. Ketamine, an anesthetic with hallucinogenic effects, is being used legally in the United States for medicinal purposes. Then–NFL player Kenny Stills told me for *Sports Illustrated* that he has taken ketamine in a controlled medical setting—and did so during his playing career, too.

Stills, who has experienced depression, used ketamine once through a company called Field Trip, whose founder, Ronan Levy, I spoke to for *Sports Illustrated*. He was cleared by a psychiatric screening before being allowed to trip (people with certain conditions, like bipolar disorder and borderline personality disorder, aren't typically considered a good fit for psychedelic-assisted treatment). Despite Carcillo's experience with a microdosing regimen, many experts say effective therapy actually requires high doses.

Stills wore headphones and eyeshades and was accompanied by a therapist at all times. At one point, he called her over to hold his hand so he could feel more grounded. Stills also talked to her while tripping so she could write down what he was seeing. They processed it afterward. So what do athletes actually see when they're tripping? Of course, it varies. I'm not so interested in recapping the details of their visions. To me, to get swept up in these stories of and about tripping is to lose the point, like someone painstakingly describing a particularly wacky dream. To the people experiencing them, they can be extremely serious and meaningful, but they're not the end goal. (I should probably say that I've never tried psychedelics. At least one of my sources has urged me to. My bipolar self will pass.)

"It's not about going out and getting blasted and having a crazy trip and seeing crazy colors," said Evans, who has taken toad and psilocybin in the years since he retired. "That's something that can happen, but that's not where it's at. The true goal in all of this is perspective." In other words, it's what comes afterward and its potential to heal old wounds. It also makes some people feel at peace with themselves.

Aside from ketamine, if you take a look at the currently illegal psychedelics (as of early 2023), research for MDMA, also known as ecstasy, is the furthest along and also the closest to full Food and Drug Administration (FDA) approval. It's been studied primarily to treat people with PTSD, which is especially common among athletes. Multidisciplinary Association for Psychedelics Studies chief scientific officer Berra Yazar-Klosinski told me for *Sports Illustrated* that research has had promising results. According to interviews conducted by independent clinicians not involved in the patients' treatment, daylong therapy sessions people with PTSD have after taking MDMA are more effective than both daylong sessions without MDMA and traditional (60- to 90-minute) talk therapy sessions. Athletes have been included in those studies. (A 2023 *Wired* report suggested that much more research needs to be done to ensure that the therapy part of psychedelic-assisted therapy is appropriate, regulated, and effective.)

That's a pretty big deal. Carcillo, who founded the life-science company Wesana Health, is also counting on FDA approval—for psilocybin clinical trials on people with traumatic brain injuries. That drug, of all the psychedelics, so far has the best evidence of treating people with major depression and addiction. Carcillo's goal is to develop a holistic wellness treatment program that includes magic mushrooms. Outside of clinical trials, it seems, it will still be a while before athletes are regularly using psychedelics to treat mental illnesses and traumatic brain injuries. Could leagues run clinical trials themselves? They sure could, and I think it's something executives should be exploring.

I don't know whether most leagues have done their research—I suspect not—but running psychedelic clinical trials is something the UFC has considered doing in partnership with Johns Hopkins. Jeff Novitzky, the outfit's senior vice president of athletic health and performance, told me for *Sports Illustrated* that he started looking into it in late 2020, after HBO aired a *Real Sports* episode on psychedelics in athletes, featuring Carcillo and others. He's fielded many questions from fighters curious about the medicines, particularly psilocybin.

While Novitzky ultimately decided against pursuing clinical trials for now, in part due to concern over the ethics of administering a placebo to someone who may really need psychiatric help, he hasn't ruled it out for the future. "We're not going to sit back and wait for 10 or 20 years and see things develop without trying to find some solutions to mental health early on," he told me for *Sports Illustrated*. "We're not afraid of new things."[16] Evans also thinks UFC will circle back to the idea. It's fear, he said, that keeps other sporting bodies away.

* * *

It would be tough to write about psychedelics in sports without at least mentioning longtime Green Bay Packers quarterback Aaron Rodgers (now a New York Jet), at the time of writing easily the most famous athlete on the planet who has said they've used psychedelics. In August 2022, he joined his friend Aubrey Marcus on a podcast episode to discuss, for the first time, his use of ayahuasca. "To me, one of the core tenets of your mental health is that of self-love," Rodgers said. "That's what ayahuasca did for me, was help me see how to unconditionally love myself.

It's only in that unconditional self-love, that then I'm able to truly be able to unconditionally love others. And what better way to work on my mental health than to have an experience like that?"[17]

There's an important distinction to draw, though, between an experience like Stills's (who was previously thought to be the only then-current professional athlete vocal about his psychedelic use) and Rodgers's, which took place as part of a ceremony in Peru. When I spoke to Rodgers later that month, he confirmed for me that he's never taken ayahuasca (or psilocybin, which he has also tried) in a clinical mental health setting in the United States. "A lot of people have asked a lot of questions in the vein of, 'You seem so much happier and enjoying things a little bit more—what's the difference?'" Rodgers told me for *Sports Illustrated*. He was describing the change for the better his life since the pandemic hit the United States. "Doing ayahuasca was a big part."[18]

Rodgers also told me that "of course" he knew of other athletes in major professional leagues who have used psychedelics. The NFL explicitly said it wouldn't penalize Rodgers for his disclosure. In fact, experts and athletes I spoke to told me they thought that many psychedelics aren't labeled as specifically off limits by many men's and women's professional leagues. But when I reached out to the major ones for *Sports Illustrated*, only the NBA and MLB responded. The former bans ketamine, LSD, and MDMA. Same for the latter, which also prohibits ayahuasca, psilocybin, and mescaline. WADA bans MDMA from use in competition. It doesn't mention other psychedelics. McDuff told me that the likelihood of athletes using psychedelics at this point is low enough that leagues and governing bodies likely aren't developing costly urine tests that can even detect them. Symonds quipped that the Women's Premier League, where she played rugby, doesn't "have money to drug test us."

Both Stills and Jake Plummer, an NFL quarterback who retired in 2007, think it's time for leagues like the NFL to actively look into the potential benefits of psychedelics as the UFC did. Plummer, who now makes a living of farming non-psychedelic mushrooms, told me he talked to Rodgers before his 2022 podcast appearance and appreciated the superstar's openness. He said that he himself became familiar with magic mushrooms at a young age due to people in his close circle.

Psychedelics, Plummer said, "take you to a new place that connects you with nature, that connect you back to the belief that we're all one, we're all together, and every moment is precious." He, like others I spoke with, is quick to remind me that psychedelic revelations don't tend to do much if you don't have a plan for afterward to integrate your findings into your daily life. One of Plummer's business partners once told him something to the effect of, "You can go 30 years and see a psychologist and talk everything out week to week to week, or you can go get a two-by-four of psilocybin upside the head and get a lot of realizations."

After retiring from the NFL, Plummer said he experienced depression. "When I left, I really wanted to get away from everything. I just wanted to go where I could and not have to be Jake 'The Snake' Plummer and answering questions and signing autographs, taking pictures," he said. "I'm still this guy that did this, that played this game, but deep down, who am I?" He had to fight through the toxic masculinity—his words—that football breeds. He also had a rough time recovering from hip surgeries. In addition, he even saw fellow NFL veterans killing themselves—most notably 1990s all-decade linebacker Junior Seau in 2012. Seau was found to have CTE, which has affected scores of other football players. "A lot of guys come out of [football] a shell of themselves," Plummer said.

More than anything, Plummer wants to show the NFL's commissioner the retreats and ceremonies he said already happen in the offseasons with players and former players. "Maybe it's time to step in front of this and not be scared to lead," said Plummer, who has taken psilocybin, ayahuasca, and peyote. "There's lots of healing to be done."

There are, of course, few easy answers when it comes to substances and what might help or harm an athlete. Experts would agree that alcohol use can often be detrimental to an athlete's mental health. Opiates, too. But what about something like cannabis, which isn't so clear-cut? And what about psychedelics? It's hard to know, and experts like Walton and Johnson said we're a ways away from elite athletes using them en masse outside of clinical trials. But that doesn't mean they can't be useful data points.

"We're in a mental health crisis," Johnson told me for *Sports Illustrated*. "So hey, we need to explore it all. We need to have more options if it can be done with safety and efficacy. While some people might be against traditional medications, I'm certainly not. I'm more in the category of looking for something that can work better for more people." In the end, that's all we can do, right? Better to muddle through a host of different, imperfect solutions than to not try at all.

Chapter 9

Body Image

Eating Disorders in Professional Athletes

U.S. ALPINE SKI RACER ALICE MERRYWEATHER HAS LIVED WHAT SOME would consider a dream during her seasons abroad. "We just go from hotel to hotel and eat rich foods at European restaurants," she said. But her self-talk each year, especially around the end of the season, got worse: "Oh, I don't look like an athlete," the 2018 Olympian would tell herself. "I just put on fat all winter."

Near the end of March 2020, as lockdown for the coronavirus pandemic began in the United States and Merryweather shouldered a heavy course load at Dartmouth, her body image–related self-doubt and self-loathing intensified. In turn, her stress levels ramped up. She began restricting her diet. "I decided that gluten made me feel poorly and dairy made me feel poorly," Merryweather said. There was a level of truth to that because she had experienced some stomach problems, but she didn't replace what she was cutting, nutritionally speaking. "The patterns and the pathways in my brain very quickly turned food into a fear," she added.

Her boyfriend, who she was living with, put her symptoms—the way she was acting around food, her talk about her body, her mood swings—into Google. It came up as an eating disorder, Merryweather said. "I kind of laughed him off at that point," she added. "No, I wouldn't have an eating disorder. . . . I'm an alpine skier. That's not something that would happen to me."

Merryweather's coaches warned her in mid-June 2020 to make sure she was getting enough to eat after body composition testing revealed that her numbers were down for size, weight, and fat. In Europe for camp that September, everyone—including Merryweather—realized something was wrong. She was so cold on the hill that she could barely do her rounds of training. After that, she'd go hiking alone to burn calories, not to see the sights. On the last night of camp, Merryweather went to her team's physical therapist, bawling. "I just told her something was wrong," she said. "I don't know what's going on. But this has been so hard, and I'm so confused." The physical therapist hugged her and told her they'd figure it out together. It was in Texas at a hospital affiliated with the USOPC that Merryweather first heard a diagnosis for what she was going through: anorexia nervosa.

* * *

As Merryweather could tell you, even athletes who aren't involved in sports built around aesthetics or weight class are constantly weighed and measured and scrutinized and ogled. The prevalence varies by sport, but as many as 60 to 80 percent of athletes can at times struggle with eating disorders or relative energy deficiency in sport, which can develop into an eating disorder, said Rebecca McConville, a sports dietician. She specializes in eating disorders and once played basketball (guard) at Missouri Valley College, an NAIA school. Also, anorexia is the mental health diagnosis with the second-greatest mortality risk (behind opioid use), McConville said.

Of the three main types of eating disorders listed in the *DSM-5*, the most common is binge-eating disorder; followed by bulimia nervosa, which is characterized by binging and purging; less common still is anorexia nervosa. Which athletes are more at risk for eating disorders depends on which sport they play. The thinking goes that those who participate in aesthetic sports (like figure skating and gymnastics), endurance sports (running), power/strength-to-weight sports (cycling or climbing), weight-cycling sports (wrestling and combat sports, where athletes tend to alternate between losing and gaining weight), and antigravity sports (ski jumping) are at higher risk than others. Essentially, sports with any formal connection to weight can exacerbate and even encourage disordered eating or full-blown eating disorders.

All athletes could develop eating disorders, though. As Riley Nickols, a sport psychologist who specializes in eating disorders and runs a private practice in St. Louis called Mind Body Endurance, put it, "I'm trying to think of a sport that I have not worked with an athlete [in]." After pausing for a few beats, he finally offered up curling. Which is not to say, of course, that curlers aren't susceptible to eating disorders, just like any other athlete, only that Nickols hasn't yet personally encountered one.

There are other types of disordered eating, too, that don't necessarily register at a clinical level as either anorexia, bulimia, or binge eating. Orthorexia, for example, is a preoccupation with healthy or "clean" eating. Mackenzie Morse, a former Dartmouth ice hockey and rugby player, dealt with orthorexia during college. "I would sit down at a team meal and physically be incapable of eating the chicken fingers and ice cream that my teammates might have," she said. She felt she would have a panic attack if she had to eat what was presented to them. "And so basically [I'd] land with a salad and a plain chicken breast, or something that would be praised."

Her teammates sometimes teased her for being the "healthy" one; her disordered eating dangerously came to be seen as dedication. "I so strongly identified as an athlete and had this picture in my mind of what the best athlete looks like, how they behaved," Morse said. "And that was somebody who was lean and cut and physically strong and whose dedication to their sport encompassed sleep and food and overcommitting to exercise." Because she was hyperfocused on being a good athlete, in hindsight, she feels that perceived virtue covered for her disordered eating at times.

Eating disorders and disordered eating, in general, like all mental illnesses, are not a choice for athletes like Morse. As clinical sport psychologist Kate Bennett wrote in *Treating Athletes with Eating Disorders*, "Let me be perfectly clear: If mental health was a choice and eating disorders were a decision, I can guarantee that I would be out of a job."[1] Also, eating disorders can't be diagnosed by appearance alone. Athletes at what are considered "healthy" or "high" weights may restrict their eating. There's no easy way to tell.

"In the United States, it's incredibly fat-phobic, and the way that you lose weight isn't really seen as problematic," said Gracie Gold, an Olympic figure skater who's dealt with depression, anxiety, and an eating disorder. "And even just the fact that you don't have to be a certain weight to 'qualify' to have an eating disorder is very confusing to people. You can still be fat and have an eating disorder. That's how that works, in the same way that there are very slender, very lean people that don't have one."

In the flawed body mass index (BMI), it's people in the "overweight" group who have been shown to be the healthiest and live the longest, said Jennifer Carter, a counseling and sport psychologist at Ohio State University who specializes in eating disorders. Muscle weighs more than fat, so many athletes are "overweight" or "obese" by BMI standards, even though they're quite healthy. Also, BMI doesn't take into account factors like ethnicity and gender, Bennett wrote. Because eating disorders are so difficult to observe and diagnose, Bennett screens every person who enters her practice regardless of why they came in.

Preconceived notions lurk everywhere in the treatment of eating disorders. "We look at someone's body, and we decide based on the snap judgment of what they look like that they must be disciplined, hardworking, strong, accomplished, capable, and virtuous, or we decide they must be sloppy, slovenly, lazy, et cetera," said medical doctor Jennifer L. Gaudiani, who practices in Denver and specializes in eating disorders. Dr. G, as she prefers to be called, treats a lot of athletes. "It's an absolutely unacceptable bastion of stigma that unfortunately remains acceptable across the entire political spectrum, where people still feel that it is acceptable to fat-shame someone or even to discuss weight loss [and] weight gain in positive or pejorative terms freely without any thought as to how that might harm somebody."

Anecdotally, former swimmer Amanda Beard, a seven-time Olympic medalist from the United States who has struggled with bulimia, thinks there's still more stigma around eating disorders than there is around conditions like depression and anxiety. People "put you in this little category of, 'Oh, you've had an eating disorder, you're gonna go over here,'" said Beard, who has also experienced depression and substance use. "You're like, 'Hey, you understand how many people have had issues with food and eating and their body image?'" Filmmaker and climber Caroline Treadway feels the same. "Everyone's afraid to say that they've struggled with an eating disorder, for some reason," she said. "From my perspective, I'm like, what's the big deal? Let's just talk about this. But I think some top climbers, they must be afraid to lose sponsorships. It's scary, right?"

Not even eating disorder professionals are immune to weight bias. (That might have something to do with the fact that, as one U.K. study showed in the *Postgraduate Medical Journal*, medical school students spend less than two hours of time on eating disorders.) There aren't enough trained professionals to go around who specialize in treating athletes in particular. "There are more people looking for support than there are people well trained and able and free to provide it," said Jenny Conviser, a clinical and sport psychologist who specializes in eating disorders in athletes and is an associate professor of psychiatry at Northwestern University. She was a gymnast in college and later coached the sport, giving her a holistic understanding of how mental health issues manifest in athletes. Dr. G echoed Conviser. "That disconnect is unacceptable and outrageous, so I am constantly trying to promote education and best practices, better practices, acknowledging my own biases, my own failings, and trying to sort of model how we can take the field forward," she said. Gaudiani considers herself a weight-inclusive provider.

In talking to her colleagues one day, Conviser had a hunch about how people not properly trained in eating disorder care can worsen the problem: "All we have to do is look at somebody the wrong way, and they get an eating disorder," she remembers thinking. "All we have to do is talk about a calorie, and someone's getting an eating disorder." So Conviser and other researchers did the work to investigate her suspicion, published in March 2018 in the *International Journal of Eating Disorders*. They found that, indeed, kids who have any sort of chronic illness with a food component that required seeing a dietician were at greater risk of developing eating disorders than their peers.

Conviser's point is this: "The research has been out there for 15, 20 years now that much of this focus on diet and numbers and BMI and weight and changing your body does more damage than good," she said. "But there's still a lot of it happening." Athletes, of course, are just as susceptible to misinformation and pressure as anybody else. That threatens not only their physical health but their mental and emotional health as well.

Among athletes and those who root for them, Carter thinks another big misconception is that changing someone's weight—whether increasing or decreasing—will automatically improve their performance. There's also the matter of perfectionism. It's found in both high-achieving athletes *and* in athletes with eating disorders (not two mutually exclusive groups). "The very same factors that make them incredibly successful athletes also can give them incredibly strong eating disorders," said Natasha Trujillo, the primary therapist at Athlete EDGE, an athlete-specific eating disorder treatment program at the Denver-based center EDCare. She played basketball growing up, with intentions to compete at the Division I level before injuries derailed her.

For Beard, bulimia was about exerting control over her body when other areas of her life were spinning out of control. "It was this weird way of making myself feel better, for all these other things are going on outside in my life that I couldn't control or take care of," she said. "So I was really just focused on, okay, well, I don't like my body. I don't think it looks good. It's bad. So I'm gonna really scrutinize every single thing that I'm putting into my body and how my body looks. I'm going to weigh myself all the time. I'm gonna just obsess over it, really."

* * *

There are tons of risk factors for eating disorders for anybody, even more for those who are athletes. And in athletes, medical concerns are often overlooked and accepted as the norm. The risk factors everyone can face are genetic predispositions, temperament, relationship stress, trauma, identity confusion, maturational fears, body dissatisfaction, effects of media, life transition, cultural influences, a family history of eating disorders, and a history of controlling nutritional intake.

The athlete-specific risk factors include coach–athlete relationships, team dynamics, revealing uniforms, and season status (athletes are at highest risk during the offseason, away from their support systems). Others are performance level, injuries and other interruptions of training, starting sports early in life, overtraining, weight cycling, and sport type. Importantly, athletes who develop eating disorders can fall into one of two buckets: those whose mental illness is directly connected to their sport and those whose mental illness developed completely independently of their sport.

Additionally, most people think of eating disorders and picture wealthy, white, cisgender, heterosexual women. Statistically, imagining a woman might make sense: Among the general population, eight out of 10 people who seek treatment for anorexia or bulimia are female. And for binge-eating disorder, six out of 10 are female. Similar numbers hold true among the athlete population, Carter said. And girls and women have extra risk factors to contend with. Take revealing uniforms. For example, in beach volleyball, "Do the women *need* to wear these tiny bikinis?" Carter asked. "What is that about, versus the men are wearing tank tops and shorts?"

But the reality is anyone can have an eating disorder, and our stereotypical image of a woman can leave people who don't fit the majority's mold suffering in the shadows. "I think it's hard for men because eating disorders are seen as a female disorder," Carter said. "And they're a human disorder. You know, we all have to eat."

Treadway, the climber, made a 2021 documentary called *Light*, in which she examines the pervasive issue of often-undiagnosed eating disorders and disordered eating in climbing as well as her own experiences with anorexia and bulimia growing up before she started in the sport. Because almost no men would agree to talk to her on camera for the film, she was surprised to see that her audience for the movie skewed male. She has also noticed that men in climbing seem more likely than others to fat-shame their peers. "Guys are like, 'Oh, you fat fuck,'" Treadway said.

For men with eating disorders, it can be hard to even recognize something's wrong. Mike Marjama played catcher briefly for the Seattle Mariners in 2017 and 2018. He was formally diagnosed with anorexia and bulimia in high school but contended there were "a lifetime of events and experiences that led into it." He wanted to get girls. "I remember Abercrombie was big back in the day, and everyone carrying around those bags," he said. "Girls adored the guys on the bags, and I was like, *Oh, I just want to be that guy*." Because he was a boy, he didn't think eating disorders were for him. "When someone says 'eating disorder,' you're like, 'Oh, I'm a dude. I don't have that issue. I just want to have a six-pack.'"

U.S. Olympic figure skater Adam Rippon never felt like he had disordered eating, either, because he never thought he had body image issues. "I was fine," he said, recalling his earlier thinking. "I just didn't eat a lot. I would feel hungry, but I would push past that, and I'd be like, 'This is just what it takes.'"

In 2018, Rippon became the first openly gay athlete to medal at the Winter Olympics, earning a team bronze medal in figure skating in PyeongChang. His wake-up call came a year before those Games, when he broke his foot. He didn't break it on the ice; rather, he hurt himself running at the rink before lacing up his skates. He did a few small jumps and heard a crack. "It was in those next few weeks and those next few months that I really thought about [how] I haven't been feeding my body," he said. "I wouldn't have had this injury had I been having calcium—had I been focusing on being as healthy as possible instead of being as small as possible."

Although Rippon might have realized in 2017 that he had a problem, he still had years of struggle ahead. In retirement after the Olympics, he felt lazy for eating a regular diet while no longer pushing himself to his athletic extremes on the ice. He'd drink coffee in the morning without eating anything for days at a time and call it "finding a balance" with days when he ate more. "[Today,] it's really hard for me to enjoy food in the way that I think that a lot of people can enjoy it because of my past relationship with it," Rippon said.

Queer athletes, especially those who are nonbinary or transgender, have a significantly higher prevalence rate of eating disorders than their cisgender peers, Nickols said. In particular, Dr. G cited a study of college students that self-reported eating disorder behaviors and showed that they were about four times more prevalent in nonbinary and trans people.

Those athletes face overlapping but not identical sets of challenges in eating disorder recovery compared with other athletes. Nonbinary or transmasculine athletes, for example, may avoid restoring their weight to a healthy goal because they experience body dysmorphia associated with their menstrual cycle, which often disappears when people restrict their eating. In those cases, Bennett said, professionals should affirm athletes in their identities and introduce them to other means of eliminating the menstrual cycle, like using certain kinds of intrauterine devices.

Schuyler Bailar, a former Harvard swimmer, was the first openly trans man to compete on the men's team for an NCAA Division I school across all sports. He figured out he was trans while in residential treatment for an eating disorder (he prefers not to specify which one, as he believes that sharing specific eating disorder behaviors could be harmful to others). "A lot of trans people will report that their eating disorder takes root in their desire to control their body after or during puberty, when it begins to change in ways that feel really antithetical to who we are," Bailar said. "That definitely was an experience with mine, but it's not the same for everybody, and it's not always the sole 'cause' or root of the eating disorder."

Bailar began transitioning in 2014 after he'd recovered from his eating disorder and self-harming behaviors. That was before he attended Harvard. He described his decision to transition as "a love letter for my body." He added, "I always say that going through puberty the first time made me feel like I was growing out of my body. I was growing away from it. And when I took testosterone, I very much felt like I got to grow into my body." He also described top surgery as lifesaving.

Dr. G said, "It's all well and good for eating disorder therapists to say, 'Love your body.' But if you were not born into the right body and changing how you eat—even if it's not great for either your mind or your health—is one of the ways you stay safe in the world and can be in a body that's even tolerable, we really have to have a conversation about where pathology crosses into reasonability." Bennett added, "We have ways to support a healthy body without using the eating disorder as a way to still support that gender identity."

* * *

Once, after a summer of training in the gym, Merryweather saw her ski coach for the first time since spring. At the on-snow camp, he eyed one of her teammates and said, "You're looking really dense these days." Merryweather and her teammates all looked at each other like *uhhhhhh*. "I know he means it as a compliment, but that feels really questionable," Merryweather said. "It's things like that that seem very normalized and can seem harmless in small doses, but when you really pay attention, those comments are everywhere."

Merryweather recognizes that as an athlete, her and her teammates' bodies are going to be the subject of some conversation during training. "They're very important to be talked about, but there's a way to respect and honor the way an athlete is able to use their body instead of comparing or focusing on certain physical attributes like weights or 'oh yeah, she's incredibly muscular' or 'she's one of the larger skiers on the circuit.'"

In general, coaches' influences play a huge role in athletes' chances of developing eating disorders, whether or not they realize it. "I think a risk factor for eating disorders in sport is nonexperts making decisions about weight and nutrition," Carter said. "A lot of people think, *Well, if you just try hard enough, you can lose this weight, and then you can start eating how you were eating, and then you'll be fine.*" In reality, she said, 95 percent of people regain the weight they lost within two years, and there's no research to support the fact that an athlete needs a certain weight, BMI, or muscle mass to succeed.

Despite the lack of expertise coaches may have, athletes are conditioned to look to them for support and advice. "It's alarming because we continue to see in research that they turn to their teammates, coaches, and Google above even utilizing a dietitian if there's one on staff," McConville said. "Having coaches stay in their lane is something we're really advocating for."

A coach who means well might approach one of their athletes and say, "I want you to lose weight." To Carter, this is not an appropriate comment: "That athlete would probably lose some power if she tried to lose weight," she said. "It may not improve performance." Additionally, that athlete may already be at risk of developing an eating disorder, making the situation even more dangerous.

Nickols said he's worked with coaches who would hand athletes menus on the road with some meal choices already crossed off. When asked by Nickols what the intent was, one coach said something like, "Well, they don't need to be having chicken Alfredo." To which Nickols responded, "Well, what's wrong with chicken Alfredo? I like chicken Alfredo." Eliminating meal options because they're perceived to be "unhealthy" sends the message to athletes that they might not be dedicated enough to their sports or their bodies if they prefer foods that their coaches think aren't good for them.

As with other mental illnesses, there's also a culture of fear around athletes speaking up about eating disorders. Athletes are constantly wondering "what their coaches will know, what their coaches will not know," Trujillo said. They also ponder "how it might impact playing time or opportunities in their sport," she added, calling it a "huge factor."

In particular, coaches who don't necessarily mean well can further exacerbate that culture of fear. While training with Nike's Oregon Project coach Alberto Salazar, elite runner Mary Cain lost her menstrual period for three years and suffered five broken bones. She began to have suicidal thoughts and started cutting herself. "I was the victim of an abusive system, an abusive man," Cain said. "Alberto was constantly trying to get me to lose weight. He created an arbitrary number of 114 pounds, and he would usually weigh me in front of my teammates and publicly shame me if I wasn't hitting weight. He wanted to give me birth control pills and diuretics to lose weight—the latter of which isn't allowed in track and field."[2]

Olympic runner Kara Goucher, who also trained under Salazar, recalled teammates being weighed in front of one another. She described to the *New York Times* the fear she had opening unsanctioned energy bars in her room because perhaps an assistant coach would hear the wrapper noise. "When you're training in a program like this, you're constantly reminded how lucky you are to be there, how anyone would want to be there, and it's this weird feeling of, 'Well, then, I can't leave it. Who am I without it?'" Goucher told the paper in 2019, when Cain blew the whistle about Salazar's harmful tactics. "When someone proposes something you don't want to do, whether it's weight loss or drugs, you wonder, 'Is this what it takes? Maybe it is, and I don't want to have regrets.' Your careers are so short. You are desperate. You want to capitalize on your career, but you're not sure at what cost."[3]

Nickols sees the coaching influence on eating disorders as black and white. "I tell coaches you foster and create an environment in your team that either promotes [disordered eating] or prevents it," he said. "There's no middle ground." When coaches hear talk among teammates about body shaming or the need to do extra workouts to slim down bubbling up, Nickols recommends they step in and shut it down firmly with something like, "We're not talking about that. That has no place on this team." More education would help. "I would love for coaches and trainers and parents and athletes just to have more awareness of body image, of fueling properly for sport, of body acceptance, of dos and don'ts, like what to say, what not to say," Trujillo said.

* * *

The media and social media also play a huge role in how athletes feel about their own body image and eating habits. "It's like they're describing livestock or horses," Maria Rago, a clinical psychologist and the president of the board of directors of the National Association of Anorexia Nervosa and Associated Disorders, told the *New York Times'* Maggie Astor about the history of journalists discussing athletes' sizes.[4] Astor's article goes into detail about the 1994 death of U.S. gymnast Christy Henrich and the flawed gymnastics, overall sports, and journalistic cultures that contributed.

That was before social media. "I think Instagram glorifies a certain type of body, or what you might see on your Explore page could have nutrition information that isn't actually being provided by a certified nutritionist or dietician," Merryweather said. "There's an overflow of information and body ideals that's out there now, and that can get away from the idea of celebrating a body's accomplishments and a person's accomplishments for what a body can do and not what a body looks like."

McConville said it's not just the likes of Instagram that can be troublesome territory for athletes. They also have to be careful with apps like Strava, a fitness tracker that shares workout data via GPS with connections. "Basically at all times, there's somebody that you can compare to, image-wise and performance-wise," she said. "If their brain is always trying to strive for feedback that they are doing well, there's the playground for it."

For Beard, it wasn't just her drive for perfectionism or swimming in revealing bathing suits that gave her trouble with her bulimia. She was also modeling for magazines like *Maxim*. "They don't wanna shoot me on this photo shoot," she said, outlining her thinking at the time. "I must be fat."

Part of Merryweather's reason for coming forward about her own eating disorder while still in treatment was to decrease her own shame and see whether she might be able to help others by sharing an authentic story of struggle on social media. After posting on Instagram, she heard from "a shocking number of athletes and even ski racers who have had similar experiences," she said. "It was both very heartwarming and really sad and kind of scary to know how much suffering was going on because of eating disorders and because of the way I think athletes' bodies are spoken about, the way food is approached in the athletic world." When we spoke in 2021, Merryweather said she still considered herself to be in recovery.

Another person who knows a thing or two about the influence of the media on athlete mental health is Monica Seles, the former world No. 1 tennis player who joined the Women's Tennis Association tour on February 13, 1989, when she was barely 15. When she was 18, a reporter asked her, "Monica, are you wearing a different style of dress because your body has changed?" When she asked him to clarify, he said, "Your backside. It's gotten bigger over the last year." It was near the start of a toxic relationship between the media and her body, which she chronicled in 2009 in her autobiography *Getting a Grip: On My Body, My Mind, My Self.*

When Seles turned 19, the real trouble began. At a Hamburg, Germany, tournament on April 30, 1993, a fan who wanted Steffi Graf at the top of the rankings plunged a nine-inch serrated boning knife into Seles's left shoulder blade as she bent over to sip water during a changeover. She would later write that the trauma launched her into depression and PTSD. "There was a problem that no CAT [*sic*] scan or MRI readout could diagnose," she wrote. "Darkness had descended into my head and it was going to stay awhile. No matter how many ways I analyzed my situation, I couldn't find a bright side. I could play again? Great. Maybe I didn't even want to play again."[5]

While Seles recovered and while her father was undergoing treatment for cancer in his stomach, she secretly binged Oreos, Pop-Tarts, pretzels, and barbecue potato chips. When she returned to the court eventually, newspaper reporters during Wimbledon said she looked like a sumo wrestler, she wrote. Later, by the end of 1996, she wrote that an international newspaper had featured a photo of her tanning on the deck of a boat. The copy apparently read, "It's game, set and crash for tubby tennis champion Monica Seles who looks like she's had a serving too many during a diving holiday in the Caribbean."[6] Then at Wimbledon in 1997, she kept eyeing on newsstands a photo of all the players' butts lined up next to one another, while the public was polled on whose was best.

Seles tried seeing therapists, athletic trainers, and nutritionists. Food became, she wrote, her comfort and poison. "The bigger I got, the smaller I felt as a person," she wrote, "spinning like a neurotic hamster on the wheel of quick fixes and extreme diets."[7] Binge-eating disorder wasn't even recognized as a distinct condition until the *DSM-5* came out in 2013. Although the press did notice Seles's periodic weight gain, Bennett has warned, "People often assume that they can tell whether athletes have eating disorders based on how they look. This is a faulty assumption. Eating disorders are masters of disguise."[8] Surely, the reporters who dogged Seles throughout her career wouldn't have suspected that an athlete of her stature could struggle with an eating disorder. They were wrong.

* * *

For any eating disorder patient, there are three prongs to the treatment approach, Carter said: psychological, medical, and nutritional. Typically, the athletes she sees also meet with registered dieticians. Treatment teams may include a host of other professionals, too: a psychopharmacologic provider, a family therapist, and a movement therapist or athletic trainer (common for NCAA athletes), to name a few. The athletes themselves can choose whether their head coaches and strength and conditioning coaches are involved in the plan: They could be helpful additions, assuming that those coaches don't encourage unhealthy behaviors.

There's also the matter of choosing the level of treatment an athlete needs. Inpatient treatment is the highest level of possible care for athletes (or others) with eating disorders. The main intention is to medically stabilize the athlete. One step down is residential treatment, which is still 24-hour care, but patients have more freedom to move around throughout the day and participate in individual and group therapies, along with psychiatric and nutritional appointments. From there, steps down include partial hospitalization, where the patient spends most of their days at the hospital but sleeps at home; intensive outpatient programs; and regular outpatient programs.

Following the three-pronged approach, Merryweather started with a regular outpatient program, seeing a dietician, a sport psychologist, and a therapist who specialized in working with eating disorders. In November 2020, though, her team realized she needed a more intensive treatment system; it was simply too much for her to "rewire her pathways," as she put it, while living on her own. So she went to Denver for a six-week partial hospitalization program, where she'd spend full days at the hospital but leave in the evenings. "It ended up being some of the best six weeks of my life, in a weird way," she said.

Merryweather was lucky to have her mom by her side. She flew out right away and stayed with her daughter for the duration of the program. The first day, Merryweather came home at 6:30 p.m. crying. "I was like, 'I hate it, Mom. This is the worst,'" she said. "With a lot more expletives thrown in." She didn't feel "sick enough" to be in treatment and wasn't convinced she needed that kind of support, at least during the season, when in her mind she should've been skiing.

But at one point during Merryweather's second week of treatment, on the thirteenth floor of the hospital in a west-facing room, she basked in the afternoon sunlight in between therapy sessions. "I almost started laughing because it was such an instant rush when I felt this sunlight that I suddenly felt calm and happy and excited and hopeful," she said. "It was such a powerful emotion that it made me realize how little I'd experienced that. . . . It was really important for my recovery to realize, *Oh, I haven't felt like this in a really long time.*" It was then she knew the treatment was working.

Bailar also started with outpatient treatment but was told he needed a residential approach. He started at Oliver-Pyatt Centers in Miami the day after his high school graduation. "That place absolutely saved my life," he said.

Marjama's experience at an inpatient program in high school wasn't as happy as Merryweather's or Bailar's. "I would say you're in prison," he told me. After a couple of weeks, he was stabilized and transferred to an outpatient program.

* * *

While athletes are people first—and therefore a lot about treating an athlete with an eating disorder is the same as treating anyone else—there are key differences that experts who specialize in working with athletes take into account for those who play sports at a high level. For example, at the University of Arizona, Beard saw her campus nutritionist, who didn't seem to realize or care that she was an athlete, let alone what was doable in terms of preparing meals in her tiny dorm room, the swimmer wrote in her 2012 memoir, *In the Water They Can't See You Cry.*

In recent years, specialized, athlete-specific treatment programs have cropped up, such as the Victory Program at the treatment center McCallum Place in St. Louis, which Nickols oversaw for eight years. Now he consults for Athlete EDGE, where Trujillo works. Previously, EDCare ran a program called Elite for athletes. That was created in part by Bennett and USOPC mental health director Jessica Bartley.

One primary difference in treatment programs such as Victory and Athlete EDGE versus programs for the general population is the incorporation of exercise into recovery. "Sometimes it's taboo in more traditional eating disorder treatment centers to talk about exercise because there are a lot of people who just struggle with that. So even bringing that up in a group can be triggering for other patients," Nickols said. "But I think with athletes . . . there's safety in talking about that openly, without having to monitor what you're saying."

Not long ago, the thinking was that athletes who struggled with eating disorders shouldn't *ever* return to their sports. "There was a lot of research saying that if an athlete returns to sport, they're going to relapse, so we should just tell them to give up their sport and move on with their life," said Bennett, who has also been a competitive cyclist and cycling coach. "It wasn't okay for me to hear that because I knew that people could go through recovery and get back to life and get back to sport in a healthy way if they were very motivated."

Bennett started questioning the common wisdom in grad school and seeking out other providers and researchers who were doing the same. "Here we are, over a decade later, with a lot of research supporting yes, we can do this," Bennett said, "and a lot of evidence supporting that yes, you can go through recovery and still be a competitive athlete." It's a concept she gets challenged on occasionally. But now, programs like Victory and Athlete EDGE integrate sport training and oversight for athletes into other facets of treatment. Bailar and his father chose Oliver-Pyatt over other options because that center agreed to let him return to swimming during the second half of his five-month stay. While he knew he needed a break from his sport, being able to return to it with supervision so that he wasn't overexercising or resorting to old behaviors was key to his recovery.

McConville said she'd love to hear more stories, like that of Molly Seidel, of people who stepped away from their sport to get treatment and then returned and excelled. She's referencing the U.S. long-distance runner who took bronze in the Olympic marathon in Tokyo and has spoken out about dealing with bulimia, OCD, depression, and anxiety. "I think for many of these athletes, and this is what they've told me, is that they view it as having to give up their sport if they feel like they have that eating disorder diagnosis," McConville said. "So I love it because I think athletes now are starting to get better, centered care for them and realizing that, you know, the brain is an organ like everything else."

Dr. G will medically clear an athlete to return to their sport once their heart rate, blood sugar, and electrolyte levels are in check. They also have to have demonstrated that their physical capacity is strong enough to handle exercise—so they're not trying to compete while nursing a stress fracture, for example. She also has to sign off that they're fueling their body appropriately to maintain a good baseline and are engaging in little to no purging behaviors since those could lead to cardiac danger. They also have to be psychologically ready to return.

The group therapy sessions athletes attend at these specialized programs stand out. The athletes do integrate with general populations to focus on skills like cognitive behavioral therapy, dialectical behavioral therapy, and developing healthy relationships. But the athlete-specific sessions are safe spaces for them to talk about the issues associated with having to step away from their teams and their sports and the isolation that can accompany that. They can also have more nuanced talks about body image issues and performance issues that might arise specifically from being an athlete. They go through mental skills training. They talk about sport culture. Bennett said there's room for big questions: What does it mean to be an athlete in the public eye? How does that affect your eating disorder? How does that affect your recovery? What does it mean to have your life broadcasted on social media?

"We don't want to do a disservice by not paying attention to those things while they're in treatment and giving them the opportunity to develop adaptive and healthy ways to engage in their sport that won't lead them right back to their eating disorder when they discharge," Trujillo said. For athletes who don't have that specialized, nuanced support and have been told to just ditch their sport for good in the name of recovery, that can create a "huge existential crisis," Bennett noted, which brings us to a broader look at how athletes cope with losing access to their sport— either temporarily or even for good.

CHAPTER 10

Life Out of the Game

Injury, Absence, and Retirement

WE'VE ALL BEEN DISAPPOINTED WHEN MUCH-ANTICIPATED PLANS WERE canceled—a trip called off due to illness or a concert missed due to a deadline imposed at the last minute. But what about preparing for that vacation or concert for *years* and then being told you couldn't go? Nearly unheard of. (Well, before COVID-19 hit, anyway.) Such is the reality for elite athletes. A crisis might mean a dream career deferred at best and terminated at worst. And the cruelest part of such an interruption can be not knowing whether an absence from sports is temporary or permanent.

Athletes are often subject to extended periods of time off—typically for injury recovery, pregnancy, or personal matters. Time without sports can be traumatic. "You feel like a nobody, and all of a sudden there's no coach to say, 'Hey, to reach this goal do x, y, z.' You're on your own," said Mackenzie Morse, a former Dartmouth ice hockey and rugby player. She started a blog called *The Sideline Perspective* to chronicle her peers' experiences coping without sport. She's also the athlete outreach and engagement manager for the USOPC. "In retiring there were a lot of questions of: What is an athlete? Who is an athlete?"

For athletes, losing such an integral part of their identity, even temporarily, can be crushing, no matter the reason. "You tear an ACL [anterior cruciate ligament] or [have] some significant injury, and then you're carted off the field and forgotten," said Gary Bennett, a Virginia Tech associate athletic director as well as a clinical and sport psychologist.

"Then you're looking at seven, eight, nine months of their lives when you're going to be separated from the team, going through a difficult rehab in hopes that they'll be able to return to play. It's an upheaval about the lives that they've known and that they're comfortable with."

Bennett, who's been at the university since 2000, would know. He was a Division III pitcher and left fielder at Centre College in the late 1970s and early 1980s, after transferring from Kentucky. He dealt with substance use in school as a way of coping with stress, though he didn't have the vocabulary and the resources around him to get proper help at the time.

There's a comparison for getting injured or otherwise stepping away from sport that may sound dramatic but rings true for many athletes and experts: "It can really mimic the grief and loss process that people experience when they lose a loved one," Kensa Gunter told me for *Sports Illustrated* near the start of the pandemic.[1] She's a licensed clinical and sport psychologist in Atlanta who also serves on the USOPC's mental health task force, formed in February 2020. Greg Harden, a former executive associate athletic director and director of athletic counseling for the University of Michigan who has worked with Tom Brady and Michael Phelps, has drawn the same comparison as Gunter did: "There's a tremendous sense of loss. It's like losing a loved one, when you take sports away," he said. "Because sports may have been the stabilizing force in my universe."[2]

Meadowlark Media's Kate Fagan distinctly remembers losing in the first round of the NCAA basketball tournament in 2004, her senior year, ending her college career. Even though she'd go on to play semipro ball for a few years, no longer suiting up for the University of Colorado Boulder felt like the end of an era. "I just remember walking around campus and just feeling like I didn't know who I was anymore," she said. While on the team, she had daydreamed about alternatives. "As I walked across the quad to practice and everyone is out there—first glimmer of spring with blankets laid out—I wanted to be those people with nothing to do. But then when I actually had it, I realized that's not what I wanted. Then there was just this really difficult melancholia I would wake up with for years."

Kelsey Neumann had similar struggles with her identity. She played for the Buffalo Beauts of the Premier Hockey Federation (then the National Women's Hockey League [NWHL]) until 2021. In the middle of her playing days, though, she had left the Beauts and tried to catch on with the competing Canadian Women's Hockey League. After getting drafted by Montreal, she drove all the way up there and paid for a hotel room on her own dime just to be told after a skate that the team wasn't seriously considering giving her a spot. She ended up taking that 2018–2019 season off before returning to the NWHL and the Beauts, seizing the chance to nurse a muscular injury in her hip. The time away from the ice, she said, was a "wake-up year." She described her internal struggle: "I grew up being Kelsey Neumann, the hockey player; Kelsey Neumann, the athlete; Kelsey Neumann, the goalie. Then who is Kelsey Neumann?"

Stepping away from the pro game helped her discover who she was without her playing career. She finally started to internalize that hockey is a part of her, not her entire being. Neumann still took coaching gigs, bolstering her experience and helping young kids grow the game, goals she pursues in conjunction with her day job as a teacher. And as for her retirement, "All roads lead to beer league," she said, perhaps not even half joking.

Even for those of us who don't play sports at the elite level, periods following injuries or other time off from recreational exercise can be extremely tough. For example, injured athletes, at least in the 1990s, experienced clinically significant depression six times as often as non-injured athletes. For me, sitting out of competitive running in high school for months at a time—and then leaving the sport permanently—led to long episodes of depression that nearly wrecked me. A close look at how *elite* athletes encounter, manage, and overcome injury, absence, and retirement can teach all of us—athletic or not—about how to deal with our own setbacks.

* * *

In its *Mind, Body and Sport* guide, first published in 2014, the NCAA includes for its athletes, coaches, and administrators a word of caution about taking care of one's mental health when injured. Using professional athletes' stories, it signals to schools, specialists, athletes themselves, and the general public that mental illness is increasingly important to the governing body. One case mentioned in the publication: In September 2010, Denver Broncos wide receiver Kenny McKinley was found to have died by suicide after reportedly growing despondent over a knee surgery he underwent a month before. Expecting to be sidelined for the entire season, he had apparently made comments to those around him about his uncertainty in the face of not being able to play in the NFL for a prolonged period of time. (He was also reportedly in a lot of debt, and suicide attempts stem from all manner of causes and health conditions as opposed to one single reason.)

Another case the NCAA spotlights is that of Picabo Street, the Olympic skier who crashed off course at a downhill event in March 1998, snapping her left femur and tearing a ligament in her right knee. She faced two years of recovery. "I went all the way to rock bottom," she told the *New York Times* in 2000. "I never thought I would ever experience anything like that in my life. It was a combination of the atrophying of my legs, the new scars, and feeling like a caged animal. I went from being a very physical person, a very powerful athlete, to barely having any strength to get from my room to the kitchen. You're stuck and you can't do what you normally do and it makes you crazy."[3] Street said she emerged from her depression only when she turned her energy toward what she had to be grateful for rather than the physical and mental toll of her injury. She returned to the sport in 2000 and was able to race for two more years before retiring.

That the NCAA details the potential for tragedy like McKinley's alongside the potential for recovery like Street's demonstrates its acknowledgment of the full range of risk and possibility for athletes. The association hasn't always been fond of highlighting sport's dangers and weaknesses for college athletes, so the move was significant, showing that mental health may be taken more seriously. Both Street and McKinley faced injury and the accompanying uncertainty but with vastly different outcomes. All athletes are likely to experience injury or other time away, like Neumann did, at some point in their careers, but no two cases are created equal. Neither are the reactions to them.

* * *

Denial, anger, bargaining, depression, and acceptance: the five stages of dying, if you ask pioneering psychiatrist Elisabeth Kübler-Ross. The model, which critics say was not empirically vetted, has long been used to apply to *grieving*, not just death, since its introduction in the 1969 book *On Death and Dying*. Grief, if researchers have learned anything since that model's debut, is not a universal experience, but many people do find their ways through some or all of those five stages.

Athletes grieving injuries and the loss of their sports are no different. While there's no one cognitive, emotional, and behavioral path to recovery and resumption of play, in 1998 a group of kinesiology and sports medicine researchers from the University of Minnesota and the Mayo Clinic developed an "integrated model of response to sports injury" in the *Journal of Applied Sport Psychology*.[4] The model outlines the interconnected responses of cognitive appraisal (what an athlete thinks about an injury and its relation to their life), emotional response (their mood and how they feel about the injury and the future), and behavioral response (how an athlete responds to injury, from planning to execution). Of course, personal factors (personality, demographics, self-motivation) and situational factors (level of competition, teammates' influence, rehab environment) also come into play.

Similar to the way we are now increasingly aware of the insidious messages of "diet culture" embedded in our society, this research posits that athletes must be conscious of the "ethic of sport," meaning the culture around athletics that encourages those injured to seek support only from their sport-related bubbles and to view injury as a necessary price to pay for competing.

* * *

Although professional athletes' stories of injury vary as much as their outcomes, the ones we hear about most generally share a common trajectory: the heartbreaking moment of onset, which is followed by a period of great uncertainty, which is then followed by an extreme showing of perseverance. But how do star athletes navigate from despair to somehow arrive there?

Breanna Stewart ruptured her right Achilles tendon while playing abroad in April 2019, just before the start of a much-anticipated WNBA season. Her domestic team, the Seattle Storm, was going to try to run it back for another title. The injury added her to the long line of basketball stars to sustain the devastating, notoriously hard-to-recover-from ailment: Kobe Bryant, Tamika Catchings, and Kevin Durant, to name a few. But Stewart wasn't prepared for a long layoff from basketball, telling the *Seattle Times* in September 2019 that she wasn't ready for the depression that set in during her rehabilitation. "It was hard to be away from [basketball] and also not be able to move," she said. "I remember always wondering, *Why is this happening? Why does this hurt? Why? Why? Why? Why? Why?* And you don't know why." (That *Seattle Times* headline, by the way? "Despite Challenges of Rehab, Storm Star Breanna Stewart Thinks She Can Be Better Than Ever."[5] Turns out she was right.)

No one is immune. Not a star WNBA power forward or even tennis legend Serena Williams. Months after Williams cut her foot on broken glass in July 2010 and endured two surgeries to repair a damaged tendon, she developed a pulmonary embolism that traveled from her legs to her lungs. She underwent yet another surgery to remove a hematoma, apparently the size of a grapefruit, from her stomach. "I definitely have not been happy," Williams told *USA Today* at the time. "Especially when I had that second surgery [on my foot], I was definitely depressed. I cried all the time. I was miserable to be around."[6] She eventually, of course, made it back to the court, as dominant as ever. During her depression, she relied on her parents and her faith to get through—and a newfound karaoke hobby. (Rihanna, Celine Dion, and Bryan Adams were her go-tos.)

As a solo athlete, Williams likely faced an even tougher challenge than her peers on teams. Sport psychologist William Wiener told *U.S. News & World Report* in 2014 that athletes who get hurt in individual sports, such as tennis or gymnastics, may be at even greater psychological risk than their peers in team sports. "Injured athletes on teams can at times be very much a part of the team and remain integrated socially, and feel engaged and invested in their team's success."[7]

* * *

Emet Marwell wasn't injured, but he realized he had no choice but to step away from his sport of choice early on in his collegiate career. While going through a major emotional upheaval, the student at Division III Mount Holyoke, a historically women's college, had to choose between being himself—transitioning genders—or continuing to play the traditionally women's sport he loved. Since high school, he had experienced anxiety and depression as part of what would later be diagnosed as bipolar II disorder. Amid the struggles, Marwell had made field hockey his world, playing for his high school team in the Washington, D.C., area. He supplemented that with skills clinics year-round to make up for getting into his sport so late.

"Field hockey was my outlet and my happy place," said Marwell, who now works as the policy and programs manager at the LGBTQ sports advocacy group Athlete Ally. He was too depressed to attend high school a lot of the time, so he watched two movies on repeat: *Silver Linings Playbook* and *Stick It*. At some points, he even got too depressed for field hockey, leading to fights with his mom over why she was paying for it in the first place.

Marwell began seriously wrestling with questions about his gender in high school. He was presenting as a "sporty jock tomboy girl" but wondering whether he could live his life as a man one day. "Is that me? Does that fit me?" he asked himself. He pushed aside that nagging feeling to pursue field hockey in college, something he never thought he'd get the chance to do. Marwell deferred a semester due to his poor mental health, including self-harm and planning for suicide. Then at college, he quickly found that being in a women's team environment was damaging his health even further. Every day at practice, he'd hear, "Here we go, ladies," and "Let's do this, girls." It grated on him.

Marwell eventually decided that for him, medical transition was the right solution. It was "so liberating and relieving but really terrifying at the same time," he said. "It took a weight off my shoulders and was really powerful to just step into my true self. And at the same time losing field hockey—I would say field hockey was another piece of my true self." Marwell wasn't allowed to continue playing women's field hockey while transitioning medically, and there is no men's NCAA field hockey equivalent.

For someone who had always identified as an athlete, Marwell felt that part of him was gone in the trade-off. He eventually found peace and joy in becoming the team manager, even attending team dinners and participating in the secret gift exchange. He also found community via Instagram with other transmasculine athletes, many of whom he noticed also struggled with mental illness and substance use. Marwell has since found his way back to sports: He now cycles for fun. "Once an athlete, always an athlete," he said.

* * *

Adam Rippon didn't think he'd have any issues retiring from figure skating after the 2018 Olympics in PyeongChang. "I was wrong," he said, laughing. He had no idea it would take him two and a half years to figure out what was wrong exactly and get those issues fixed. In the meantime, he went through periods of depression.

As an athlete, he had been wary of working with a mental performance coach or clinical psychologist. It was partially a financial issue for Rippon. "It felt like, 'Listen, do I wanna have like a little extra money so that if my tire goes flat, I can replace it?'" he said. "'Or do I wanna talk to somebody about how I'm feeling?'" And as an individual athlete, he didn't trust anybody the USOPC provided because he knew those professionals were also working with his competitors. "I would just lie, lie, lie through my teeth," telling people he'd "never been better."

In retirement, Rippon also initially steered clear of professional help. *I'm just not going to be weak*, he told himself. But he had a breakdown and finally reached out to a psychiatrist, receiving diagnoses of anxiety, depression, and attention deficit disorder. His husband and family were supportive. He slowly began to reintroduce exercise into his life and reconnect with the friends whose messages went unanswered while he was depressed. He lifts weights about three times a week in a private gym attached to the rink he used to work at. Once in a while, he skates. Balance is key.

The USOPC is doing more now, Rippon thinks, to address athlete mental health, especially after the Games conclude. When he went to Beijing in 2022 as the coach of U.S. skater Mariah Bell, he noticed a new touch point to talk about mental well-being. In a meeting for all athletes before the Games began, he heard something he hadn't in 2018. This time, the USOPC let athletes know that there would be a psychologist available to them after the competition ended. "This is a crazy experience," Rippon said. "You wait your entire life to go on a trip that's a month long and compete, and then it's all over. And that's very mentally challenging to get over."

* * *

While athletes like Rippon and Marwell step away from sports on an individual level all the time, it's rare to see people be forced to step away en masse. When the coronavirus shut down the United States in early 2020, no one had any idea what they were in for. On March 11, then–Utah Jazz center Rudy Gobert tested positive for COVID-19—which led to the announced suspension of the NBA season. (It resumed again in July with the now-famous Orlando bubble.) Other major sports leagues soon followed with cancellations of their own. The country and the world were in disarray, and sports weren't a top priority. Meanwhile, mental health among Americans worsened across the board. About four in 10 adults reported symptoms of a depressive disorder or anxiety during the early stages of the pandemic, as opposed to one in 10 from January through June 2019, according to the Kaiser Family Foundation (KFF). By July 2020, 53 percent of adults had reported to KFF that pandemic-related worry and stress negatively impacted their mental health.

"For the longest time, I've been yelling for everyone to get swimming lessons," mental skills coach Graham Betchart said. "People were like, 'I don't know,' and then 2020 came and threw your ass right into the pool." The coronavirus rattled everyone—not just those with a history of mental illness or those who had already sought out therapy. People who had never dealt with such issues were also at risk. "All of us are likely experiencing something in the mental and emotional realm that we haven't experienced before," Gunter told me in April 2020, a month into the pandemic's U.S. lockdown.[8]

Simone Biles, hunkered down in her home in Houston with her French bulldog, Lilo, cried when she heard the Tokyo Olympics were postponed. "You have those doubts," the world's most decorated gymnast told me in April 2020. "Can my body do another year? Can *I* do another year?"[9]

Biles did decide to go to Tokyo in 2021 as a 24-year-old. Her mental health struggles there didn't come out of nowhere. After all, she had told me in 2020, "I knew mentally [social distancing] would be harder than physically, because your coaches will prepare you for your competitions whenever you need to be prepared for them," she said. "But mentally, that's a whole 'nother ball game." When a crisis derails athletes' dreams, that mounting pressure has the potential to overflow, releasing a torrent of emotions. "[People] don't get that we have anxiety, that we break down," Biles said. "They just think we're perfect."[10]

Like Biles, athletes across the world had to try to figure out how to navigate their new lives. Many are creatures of habit, with regular schedules that could entail training in the morning, napping in the afternoon, competing at night, and then watching that night's film the next day. Re-creating routines while holed up at home is crucial, Chicago White Sox sport psychologist Jeffrey Fishbein told me for *Sports Illustrated*. It can include working out or rehabbing—to the extent athletes are able to from home. But finding regular slots in a day for breathing exercises, reading and writing, Xbox with friends, or even making TikToks allows for some sense of normal in a time that's anything but, said Fishbein.

During those early days of the pandemic, Biles spent her time video chatting her teammates two or three times a week, walking her dog, and, like the rest of us, going grocery shopping. Solomon Thomas, then a San Francisco 49ers defensive end, waited for an uncertain 2020 NFL season by holing up with his parents, his girlfriend, and his pit bull, Mickey. He also packed in a lot of TV (everything from *The Office* to *Little Fires Everywhere*), texted with his therapist, and remembered to drink water. "Controlling what you can control," he said.[11]

When in doubt, it's also just fine to take a breath. "I think that's incredibly important," then–Cleveland Cavaliers power forward Kevin Love, the most vocal mental health advocate in the NBA, told *Sports Illustrated*, "especially when you are trying to be really productive and try to keep the routine." He stressed, "It is okay to do nothing. It is okay to take a day. It is okay to take a few hours to just destress and take your mind off of things."[12]

* * *

If there's a silver lining in getting injured or otherwise being forced to take a step back from the sports you love (and it's understandably often hard to see or appreciate that silver lining in the moment; I personally hate talk of silver linings *and* the film *Silver Linings Playbook*), it's that such a period presents an ideal moment to press pause and reevaluate your life and pursuits. Consider it akin to taking a gap year from school or shifting gears in any other career.

In 2019, the WNBA's Layshia Clarendon injured her ankle in a freak accident—stepping on a teammate's foot in a Connecticut Sun practice—that ended up requiring surgery and months off from the game. In late 2021, they reflected, "I'm really thankful that I was injured and had that time with my therapist because I was like holy shit, if I had retired and then had to deal with all this stuff. . . . Every person should not have an injury, but every athlete should have that space to go through and examine themselves in relation to their sport. Before they retire."

As for retirement, Clarendon suggested he might have trouble letting go of his job: "It's very different than when you're a current player, right? You get the perks and the status and the things that make it cool to be a player. I will definitely when I'm done playing be like, *Damn, do I have to change my bio?* I just wanna keep WNBA in there." She laughs, perhaps nervously.

The dawn of retirement has sometimes been referred to by researchers as "social death" for the athlete. The application of this term to sports is fraught and weighty given that it was popularized in the 1980s by sociologist Orlando Patterson to describe slavery. It might also, just like describing athletes as grieving the loss of sport, sound a touch dramatic, but in a chapter of *Sport and the Sociological Imagination*, published in 1982, sociologist Edwin Rosenberg noted, "Upon retirement, even in the best scenario, the athlete is deprived for the first time of the rewards his or her sport has showered on him or her since childhood." On top of that, Rosenberg wrote, they're likely experiencing social isolation, maybe even ostracism, from their peers.[13]

In her 2022 book *My Greatest Save*, cowritten with Wayne Coffey, U.S. women's national team soccer goalkeeper Briana Scurry, of the famous '99ers, recounted her story, mental health trials and all. The death of her father in the middle of her career hit her particularly hard. "I wasn't ready to move to Florida and start playing shuffleboard, but I was trying to come to terms with my athletic mortality," Scurry wrote. "Was it time to move on, to make sure I would not be another athlete who fools herself that it will last forever? Or was I ready to plunge back into the competitive fray?"[14]

There's that concept from Rosenberg: athletic mortality. Scurry briefly held a job at a bank, thinking she'd work her way up into more advanced finance-related roles. Soccer again came calling, but it wasn't the same. "I wanted to be Briana Scurry, and I was very, very, very, very, very razor-thin close to being Briana Scurry," she told me. "And I was fit and I was ready to go and I know I could still do it, but emotionally there was a hole in the shape of my father." In that sense, her literal grief in the form of losing her dad was compounded by the grief she felt of slowly losing her grip on her career as a world-renowned soccer player. Scurry didn't retire for good until 2010, and that was not on her terms— she sustained an in-game concussion that it would take her years to fully recover from.

Language surrounding athletic retirement as social death is echoed in other athletes' own accounts of aging, too, as sociologist Stephen Lerch showed in another chapter of *Sport and the Sociological Imagination*. He pinpointed the 1976 book *Life on the Run*, by Bill Bradley, who starred for the New York Knicks in the 1960s and 1970s. Bradley, who would go on to have a second career as a Democratic U.S. senator from New Jersey, wrote, "For the athlete who reaches thirty-five, something in him dies; not a peripheral activity but a fundamental passion. It necessarily dies. The athlete rarely recuperates. He approaches the end of his playing days the way old people approach death. He puts his finances in order. He reminisces easily. He offers advice to the young. But, the athlete differs from an old person in that he must continue living. Behind all the years of practice and all the hours of glory waits that inexorable terror of living without the game."[15]

Another example that Lerch smartly collected of an athlete referencing the end of careers in sports as though they were the end of their lives came from MLB pitcher Jim Bouton in his 1970 book, *Ball Four*, which served as a diary of the previous season. Bouton succinctly yet terrifyingly described the process of getting cut by a team: "On the Yankees the Grim Reaper was Big Pete. Once he whispered in your ear that the manager wanted to see you, you were clinically dead."[16] Clinically dead. Yikes.

There are examples in fiction, too, that illustrate the bleak prospect of athletic retirement. I was eager to speak to Anelise Chen, who wrote the 2017 novel *So Many Olympic Exertions*, which deals with in large part, to greatly oversimplify things, a former athlete struggling with her grief, her mental health, and her future in general. Chen offered up other examples of stepping away from sports that she drew inspiration from, such as the short stories "Smoke" by Michael Chabon and "A Piece of Steak" by Jack London. But finding nonfiction dealing with the subject wasn't as easy for her. When Chen was writing her own book, "I don't think anyone was really talking about mental health and sports," she said. "It was hard to find material about it, so I would find them in footnotes in books." Chen herself swam growing up, and she offered some advice about how to go about life after retirement. "You just have to retrain yourself," she said.

"You have to relearn your habits. You have to reestablish your routines. You just have to redo everything about yourself."

Michael Gervais, a high-performance sport psychologist who has worked with the Seattle Seahawks, confirmed that ending a career smoothly takes a lot of work. "The really healthy, mature, insightful, extraordinary athlete meets retirement gracefully," he said. "That's rare," he added, laughing, "because they have chipped all in at a young age to be their best or the best, all of their resources have been compounded into that place, and when that gets threatened, it is incredibly scary. . . . You help them with practices to develop perspective, practices to develop insight, practices to help them with psychological skills, to manage acute and chronic stress, and you help them to reimagine the future that they would like to build for themselves and their family. . . . If you can get ahead of that before Coach or a GM says, 'Hand me your playbook,' it's great."

With the increasing help of professionals like Gervais, settling into athletic retirement is surely easier than it once was. But it's hard to read a call to action Rosenberg wrote and not find it still relevant today: "Anticipatory adjustment to retirement, or pre-retirement planning, is both under-utilized by older workers and athletes alike. Both nonsport business and the professional sport structure have begun to endorse and/or offer pre-retirement counseling, but these efforts barely scratch the surface."[17]

As a side gig, Morse—the former Dartmouth ice hockey and rugby player—has trained athletes at her alma mater who are struggling with stepping away from sports, whether it's due to the pandemic, injury, or retirement. She describes the outlook she wants to see people adopt: "So if we're looking at a challenge and our current inner voice says, *I can't, I don't know how*, etc., can we shift that to *I've done something hard before, I can take this day by day, I will show up with my best, and that's good enough?*" she asks. "Break it into something that is empowering." Any rest period, even a forced one, is an opportunity to recalibrate priorities and determine what you truly want from life.

Experts such as the White Sox's Fishbein would like to see everyone use a prolonged break from sports, be it due to injury or otherwise, to get just a little bit existential and reflect on what *really* matters in life. *"Do I need to live my life a little bit differently? Do I need to look at my own behavior?"* he said. "When we come back to sport, maybe we react to the bad game a little bit differently or the missed putt a little bit differently."[18]

After all, sports—even on the elite level—are supposed to be fun and entertaining. When we value them at the expense of our mental health, we lose the plot. Stories of so many athletes show that it's both normal to struggle and possible to thrive even while temporarily or permanently sidelined, without access to their sports. There's a lesson in there for all of us about seeking help, leaning on others, and maintaining strong routines rather than simply soldiering on alone. Perspective is everything.

Conclusion

So What's Next?

WHEN I SPOKE TO FORMER PROFESSIONAL RUGBY PLAYER ANNA Symonds in 2022, she told me something key: "We *are* the sport," she said, meaning athletes. "There's no sport without our bodies out there." Are those athletes happy? Symonds isn't so sure. She implored me to think about what keeps athletes healthy versus simply responding to illnesses and injuries like Whac-A-Mole. I had asked Symonds what I've asked nearly everyone I've talked to for this book: What do you want the future of mental health care—and the conversation surrounding it—to look like for athletes?

It's a question Mac Morse, the former Dartmouth ice hockey and rugby player I interviewed, first posed to herself. I had asked her at the end of a long conversation in 2021 what we hadn't touched on that she'd like to add.

"We talked a lot about reflection on the past, and where sports have come from, and where I've come from, and where we are now," Morse said. Then she proceeded to outline what she wanted the *future* of elite athlete mental health to look like. "Everybody's doubled down on what it means to try to be successful in sport. The idea of taking the foot off the gas pedal might seem really counterintuitive to people, but it could be the thing that we actually need right now in order to make sports sustainable for the next decade and for the next generation of athletes coming up."

In other words, Morse wants athletes to relax as much as they can and take steps back from competition when they need to. That's not just increasingly okay, but also necessary. Symonds's answer struck me just like Morse's did. Sports, Symonds was saying, are about "the intensity of being alive." So don't we want our elite athletes to not only live, but also thrive? How can we best ensure that going forward? I don't pretend to have all the answers to such a challenging question, but I'll lay out a few recommendations.

INCREASE PLAYER RESOURCES

One of the most important areas for improvement in elite sports is, quite obviously, money and resources. We've seen that more and more pro leagues are requiring mental health professionals on each team's staff—usually clinical psychologists or mental performance coaches—in addition to team doctors and trainers. Teams and leagues increasingly provide athletes with free online therapy apps and services. The science isn't totally settled as to how helpful they can be in comparison with in-person therapeutic support, but different approaches work for different people, so having more options (especially private ones) is always better. Some teams have psychiatrists at their disposal, too. Collective bargaining agreements between leagues and players' unions can ensure the continuity and strength of those resources.

On the amateur level, the USOPC's director of mental health services and her team have made strides toward meeting the increasing and reasonable demands of their athletes. Stars like Michael Phelps stress that the USOPC hasn't gone far enough. I think that's a fair criticism. It's important to keep investing money, hiring more providers, and covering more of athletes' mental health expenses into retirement. The NCAA, too, is on the right track but can go much further. Currently, the organization does not require every member institution to have a single licensed mental health provider on staff. Instead, it's simply a guideline, and schools ranging from Division I to Division III have wildly different resources at their disposal. A more concrete requirement to level the playing field is sorely needed.

Look no further than the case of Briana Scurry to understand what needs to continue to change at all levels. The U.S. women's national team soccer great got misdiagnosed "left and right," in her words, after sustaining a season-ending concussion in game action during the 2010 club campaign of the Washington Freedom, of Women's Professional Soccer (a precursor to the NWSL). Scurry retired that year, and the league formally folded two years later. She had little money and no continuing health care coverage, as she chronicled in her book with Wayne Coffey, *My Greatest Save*. In the absence of other institutional support, she filed for workers' compensation in Maryland, where her team had been based.

It took Scurry—who struggled with not only her physical symptoms, but also depression, substance use, and suicidal thoughts—years and years to get healthy. "Some days I would wake up and feel a glimmer of hope, and my old upbeat worldview," she wrote. "Other times the gloom hung so heavily over me I was sure it would never lift. I could never pinpoint what caused the depression to lighten, or what made it hit me like a tsunami."[1] At one point, she found the right doctor to treat her traumatic brain injury but needed to wait about *nine* months to get approval from the court system just to see him. A suicidal person, needless to say, doesn't always have nine months left. Scurry was nothing but a number in the workers' comp system, as she saw it.

"Everything there was deny, deny, deny," she told me in 2022. "I literally had to keep going to court to fight them to go one step ahead and then the next step. I had to fight them to get a second opinion, and then I had to actually go see [the court system's recommended] doctor first, and then I had to get that second opinion, and then I had to fight to do what the second opinion suggested." Cutting out those battles would've made a great chunk of Scurry's life significantly easier and healthier. Future generations of athletes should be taken care of better financially.

Don't Forget Coaches

Taking care of athletes' mental health isn't *only* about pouring the necessary money and resources into their care. We also need to take care of teams' and leagues' coaches and staff. They, of course, are not immune to mental illness; one Australian study conducted in 2020 found that 40 percent of elite-level coaches and high-performance support staff have experienced mental health–related symptoms, a level comparable to that of previously studied elite-level athletes. The more we can take care of those athletes' support systems, the better equipped those support systems will be, you can imagine, to take care of the athletes in their charge.

"I think a lot of times we would say, well, the mental performance coach is there to support the players. But coaches need help, too," said Ben Freakley, a sport and performance coach who has worked with teams like MLB's Toronto Blue Jays. "When I was a college soccer coach, I would've loved to be able to have somebody that I trusted to talk to about the team, about my staff, about any insecurities that I faced."

Back in 2018, as DeMar DeRozan and Kevin Love were reigniting the conversation about mental health in the NBA, Miami Heat coach Erik Spoelstra suggested that coaches would be the next focus, after players. "I'm glad the discussion of mental health now with the players is out there," he told the *Palm Beach Post*. "This is something that also relates to coaches. I've talked about it with our team. I'm glad this is starting to get to the forefront now as well because all of us need to be extremely more mindful of all the demands and how we're taking care of ourselves."[2] Unfortunately, as of this writing in early 2023, I don't think we're quite there yet.

Case in point: Former Northwestern basketball player Joanne P. McCallie spent 28 years as a head coach in the women's game at an elite level, ending her career at Duke coaching alongside men's basketball coaching legend Mike Krzyzewski (who would retire not long after her). For most of that time, she had been diagnosed with bipolar disorder. "If you are a former athlete, you especially believe that your body is sacred. Your body is strong," she wrote in her 2021 book, *Secret Warrior*. "There were times when I felt that if I could not be myself with my normal brain, then why would I want to be on this earth? I would be an imposter."[3] It wasn't until after she retired, in 2020, that she finally came forward publicly about living with mental illness.

McCallie, who was hospitalized a couple of times during the worst stretches of her bipolar disorder—once early on in her career and once after retiring—had pondered filling people in during her stint at Michigan State, but she said she was counseled by "an elder" to stay quiet. "If you do [speak up], it will always be about you," said McCallie, explaining that person's reasoning. "It will never be about the kids anymore, no matter where you win, no matter how you lose. At press conferences, there's always going to be questions: 'How are you feeling, Coach? What was that all about?' Because people try to think they understand these things, right? They think they're some kind of scientist."

So McCallie stayed quiet to focus on her players. But it shouldn't have to be like that. A coach, if they so choose, should feel free to speak up—and get support—without taking the spotlight off their players and, by extension, the mental wellness of those players. And that need for healthy athlete supporting casts goes for front offices, too.

Kalen Jackson, an owner and vice chair of the NFL's Indianapolis Colts, realized during the COVID-19 pandemic, as people everywhere were struggling physically and mentally, that she needed to put a greater emphasis on her front-office staff's mental health. When the Colts launched the Kicking the Stigma mental health advocacy campaign in 2020, it wasn't just about the players on the field. It was about everyone behind the scenes, too. Seventeen available Zoom sessions with the team clinician booked up in under 12 hours, Jackson said. Having experienced anxiety, she knew she needed to do more. She and her family of owners put in place an employee assistance program, which Jackson told me is still underused. As of our talk in late 2022, she was looking into bringing on an in-house clinician specifically for front-office staff. I haven't heard of a team employing a dedicated mental health professional for its front office before, but I think it's a great idea.

START WHEN THEY'RE YOUNG

Another way of caring for elite athletes' mental health? Make sure you *start* caring about it when they're young—before they're elite. For all the resources collegiate and professional athletes might still be lacking, kids lack even more. Few families have access to or can afford a mental performance coach, and it's not like their travel or rec teams are typically using one.

More and more, there's pressure on young kids to "specialize" in one sport rather than sample many, staying involved to simply make friends, build character, and get exercise. It's tough on their bodies *and* minds. For *Sports Illustrated*, I spoke to Tyrell Terry, who retired from professional basketball in late 2022, when he was 22. "Today I decided to let go of the game that has formed a large part of my identity," began his since-deleted Instagram post announcing the change. "Something that has guided my path since I took my first steps. While I have achieved amazing accomplishments, created unforgettable memories, and made lifelong friends . . . I've also experienced the darkest times of my life."[4]

Terry told me he felt pressure growing up to focus on basketball and basketball only despite his aptitude and interest in other sports, like baseball and football. He played in the Amateur Athletic Union, a prestigious youth basketball organization. As he grew older, spending one year at Stanford and then declaring for the 2020 NBA draft, he felt his love of basketball wane. In fact, he began to resent playing due to the anxiety—everyday puking and frequent panic attacks—it caused him. That anxiety led to depression.

Of his anxiety, Terry told me, "I would always be someone who would overanalyze: *Who's my matchup? How good are they? How am I going to perform? How many people are in the crowd? What if we win? What if we lose? What does that look like? What if I go out there and shoot 0-for-15? How does that look?*"[5] What had been fun for Terry as a kid grew to consume his entire life.

Jonathan F. Katz, a clinical and sport psychologist and performance coach, confirmed for me that as a society we've gotten just a little bit out of hand with youth sports. "We had put such an emphasis on sports in our culture. It's a little problematic in terms of youth athletes and the view of what athletics could bring," he said. "I've had people call me with very young kids who've wanted to learn how to be mentally tough. There's nothing more that young kids need from their parents than just the parents to be parents and the kids to have fun."

Some current professional athletes started working with mental skills coaches like Graham Betchart when they were just teenagers. To Katz's point, the work at that age should be less intense, but introducing kids to sport psychology concepts at an early age can be helpful. "Most young people aren't begging for vegetables, but you know to give it to them and you know it'll help," said Betchart, who has also worked on the pro level with the NBA's Utah Jazz. "Then later on in their life, they're like, 'Hey, I appreciate that. It's way better than drinking soda all day.'"

Former NFL quarterback Jake Plummer has seen a trend of professional coaches working for nonprofits that serve kids—future pros or not—and teaching them about mindfulness and other qualities that foster self-improvement and mental well-being. "There's a big movement that can happen and should be happening to teach kids more about being in the moment, enjoying it now," Plummer said. "Not working necessarily to be the next LeBron James, but just being the best you can be."

The more kids who enter high school and college with the vocabulary to express their emotions and struggles, the better. They'll be prepped to make use of the sport and clinical psychology resources offered by their programs going forward and also prepared to take a step back when their sports are no longer bringing them joy.

Talking about what ails you is, after all, a common theme across this book. We've seen that more and more athletes have spoken up about their mental illness in recent years and the snowball effect those disclosures have had on other athletes and nonathletes alike. So what can be done to keep the ball rolling?

KEEP TELLING STORIES

This directive sounds overly simplistic. And as a storyteller, it's possible I'm biased. Media practitioners should focus on building deep levels of trust with athletes. You might say that's always been the focus. For some journalists, it has been. We can all do a better job, though, of really hearing athletes if they say press conferences make them anxious or they're too depressed to go to work. And we need to avoid getting caught in a standardized, rote playbook for covering mental health in sports.

"There's a continued sense of a through line being drawn, and these athletes set the stage for us. *We need to talk about [mental health] in this way.* Is that potentially limiting to the way this is being talked about?" asked Mike Delayo, a Penn State graduate student researching the rhetoric of popular culture through sport. In other words, if every disclosure starts to sound the same or is framed the same way to fans and broader audiences, people might not internalize as much from the messages. They might stop questioning their own preconceived notions of what it means to be an athlete or to idolize one—and what it means to be "mentally tough."

Like Delayo, I don't think we're in true danger of that happening yet. We've seen there's no one formula for disclosing or relaying an athlete's mental illness. It does not have to come in a *Players' Tribune*-style first-person essay. It does not have to come in a Very Serious Magazine Feature. It doesn't even have to be the main topic of a feature. It can be a short but poignant aside, a mere blip in a player's larger story.

We also need to allow space for complications and incongruence in the narratives we hear from athletes and those around them. If you're cherry-picking whose stories sound believable or authentic, you're missing the point. Anyone can experience mental illness; they don't need to be otherwise unimpeachable to earn your trust. Athletes aren't all as widely loved as Simone Biles. Take Ben Simmons, the NBA point guard who started his career with the Philadelphia 76ers. He was traded to the Brooklyn Nets in 2021–2022 after sitting out Philly's training camp and the regular season to that point. Cynical journalists and unhappy fans were quick to label Simmons's disclosure of mental health issues a financial play, a loophole to keep receiving his salary while waiting to play for a team that might be a better fit.

Maybe money played a role—I'll probably never know, and neither will you. But there's little good that can come from a star athlete labeling themselves mentally ill, so it's something I bet very few athletes lie about for fun. If you're going to support the likes of Biles and Naomi Osaka, as I wrote for *Sports Illustrated* after the Simmons trade, you ought to support him, too. "There's not an X-ray we can present to the world, being like, 'See? It's broken.' I feel like it can always leave a little guessing game of like, is this person just being dramatic? Is it really that big of a deal?" Olympic figure skater Gracie Gold said.

Journalists and fans alike also need to broaden their conception of mental illness beyond just anxiety and depression—starting with assumptions about the shape those two conditions can take. "Lots [of people] are really understanding of depression when it looks like crying, when it's after a really tragic life event, and it's just sadness. You can't get out of bed," Gold said. "But it manifests in different ways. Your ability, lack of patience, just general apathy, and it doesn't check the box of the standard symptom list, I feel like people are less understanding, less empathetic." People with mental illness aren't always outwardly sullen. They're not always likable. We don't need to take pity on them, either, Gold said: "I don't wake up every day and think, 'Oh, wow, for someone who's depressed that was really good.' It was good or it wasn't good. Or, 'For somebody with all these issues, she skated really well.'" Gold either skated well or she didn't. We shouldn't sugarcoat that.

Plus, as Gold also believes, conditions besides anxiety and depression matter just as much, even (especially!) if we're not as familiar with them. Remember Chamique Holdsclaw's bipolar disorder and Corey Hirsch's OCD? Longtime NFL player Brandon Marshall has borderline personality disorder, and Lolo Jones, the Olympic hurdler and bobsledder, has PTSD. There are plenty of other athletes out there going through similar things. We've largely succeeded in destigmatizing anxiety and depression, at least in certain circles, and it's past time to make sure we're doing the same for all mental illnesses.

STUDY HARD
Sport psychology has its roots in the classroom, both in exercise science and in psychology itself. Tons of the experts I've spoken to for this book are academics, many of whom also work with athletes regularly. It's so important to maintain and diversify sport psychology programs so that athletes and those around them can benefit from cutting-edge research.

What Robin Vealey teaches particularly intrigued me. The professor of sport psychology at the University of Miami (Ohio) spoke to me about, in addition to the importance of women in the field, the prospects for incorporating virtual reality into athletes' training. It sounds like a buzzy idea destined to be cast aside as overrated. But Vealey patiently explained to me the concept of functional equivalence and how it can revolutionize athlete visualization.

Functional equivalence means that, say, a rower will visualize their performance better while sitting up holding makeshift oars than they would just lying down in bed. Hockey players can stand up and hold a stick during visualization. The closer you feel physically to competing, the better your mental game is going to be. Imagine, Vealey told me, a World Cup environment beamed into a (my add: probably doofy-looking) helmet an athlete can wear to transport themselves to soccer's biggest stage. The crowd noise can be controlled. Athletes can then prepare for the high-stress upcoming match by essentially already being there.

Breakthroughs like functional equivalence are huge for athletes and those around them. The more academic programs where prospective coaches and sport and clinical psychologists can learn these tips in depth, the better. I am also intrigued by a graduate psychology program the University of Denver started in 2022, housed in its new Center for Sport and Human Development. Brian Gearity, who runs the master of arts in sports coaching program, and Sheila Walker, the center's founder, saw a gap between physical performance and mental health that wasn't often addressed in schools.

Walker and Gearity are focused at first on the university's own athletes and coaches but hope to spread their work to the rest of Denver and even nationally. They are particularly concerned with cultivating a space for students and faculty to do more research into coaching—a lightly regulated field for the most part. "The coach has been likened to the CEO of the team or the organization, especially at the big-time college and professional level," Gearity told me ahead of the center's launch. "If all coaches had some sort of phys ed degree I'd feel much better, but they don't. Even that's insufficient because there's not standards, ethics, and accountability built in with regulation."

In our conversation, Walker and Gearity hit on some of my arguments above, namely, about the need to decouple youth sports from the push to win and develop elite athletes at all costs as well as the need to focus on coaches' mental health. "We're laying the groundwork to bring together education and public health and sports, to tell a new story about what's possible for young people, and to change the story about what sports is and can be," Walker said. Initiatives like the Center for Sport and Human Development seem critical to learning more about and improving athletes'—and coaches'—well-being, and I hope to see even more work like it crop up at universities.

* * *

Perhaps the most important next step to advance the mental health conversation in sports is—not to get *too* cheesy—looking inside ourselves and applying the techniques and lessons we learn from athletes to our own lives. Seemingly every expert I spoke to is big on this concept. In fact, many of the mental performance coaches I've quoted also work with musicians, actors, hedge fund employees, and military members, among other professionals.

"Those of us who will never be elite athletes, there's still things inside there that we can learn and use in terms of our mental performance," said Steven C. Hayes, a clinical psychologist and a professor of behavioral health at the University of Nevada, Reno. "We have our own mental performance challenges, and maybe they're not world class, but they're challenging us. So it's going home and talking to your loved one or getting to work and really giving it your all."

Mindfulness is not something you can practice with only the end goal of shooting a ball through a hoop. Neither is asking for help when you're down. And—once you have gained the strength to help others—neither is reaching out a hand and pulling up a friend, family member, or perfect stranger, like athletes do with their teammates all the time. Athletic or not, we are *all* worthy of robust mental health.

Acknowledgments

So many people made this book possible, starting with my agent, Iris Blasi, and my editor, Christen Karniski. Thanks to everyone else at Rowman & Littlefield for your attention to detail throughout the publication process, including but not limited to Nicole Carty and Bruce Owens, the latter of whom had the distinct challenge of copyediting a copy editor. Jennifer Keishin Armstrong, whose own books I have long admired, provided the earliest edits on this book. Charlotte Goddu saved me from myself many times in the fact-checking process. Emily K. Schwartz and Sam Yadron transcribed much of the interviews. Layshia Clarendon wrote a killer foreword. Davide Barco, thank you for the gorgeous cover art. And thank you to all the athletes and experts who shared their stories with me.

A shout-out to Astoria coffee shops, namely Gossip and Coffee Cloud, for giving me the physical space to write this book whenever I got sick of my apartment. Thanks are also due to many other nonhumans: the cats whose presence and pictures got me through this process. Penelope, first and foremost. You're a good girl, and I love you. But also Teddy, Gracie, Starling, Finch, Frankie, honorary cat Tazzy, Ellie, Lucy, Rosa, Maude, and others. You know who you are.

A ton of my *Sports Illustrated* colleagues supported me endlessly, offering words of encouragement, contacts, ideas, and commiseration: Chris Almeida, Greg Bishop, Catherine Chen, Adam Duerson, Molly Geary, Mitch Goldich, Sarah Kelly, Ben Pickman, Jason Schwartz, Stephen Skalocky, and Jon Wertheim, to name a few. And, of course, Stephen Cannella and Stefanie Kaufman.

My family and friends put up with a *lot* of talk about the manuscript from its inception to publication, and only one of them repeatedly asked me how it was coming in the voice of Stewie from *Family Guy*. Mom, Dad, Gary Kliegman, and Nicola Kliegman—thank you. Fellow new authors Katie Barnes and Michael Waters fielded many panicky texts from me. A handful of other people I'm lucky enough to spend my time around virtually and in person are the Facts and the Curious trivia team, as well as Jai Broome, Rebecca Cohen, Shaina Coogan, Keegan Dunn, Darian Jefferson, Jordyn Jefferson, Zadie Jefferson, Dawnthea Price Lisco, Will Shenton, Dan Sinensky, Megan Thielking, and Katie Wells. Jordyn, I'm glad we made the choice to stay friends that one day.

NOTES

INTRODUCTION

1. Raven Saunders, Twitter post, January 2020, 12:10 p.m., https://twitter.com/GiveMe1Shot/status/1218218968944533505.

2. Raven Saunders, Twitter post, January 2020, 12:53 p.m, https://twitter.com/GiveMe1Shot/status/1218229908171739136.

3. Alex Azzi, "Raven Saunders Opens Up about Mother's Death, Managing Grief," *NBC Sports*, 2021, https://onherturf.nbcsports.com/2021/12/09/raven-saunders-opens-up-about-mothers-death-managing-grief (February 25, 2023).

4. Tim Layden, "Michael Phelps Supports Tokyo Postponement, but Also Worries about Athletes' Depression," *NBC Sports*, 2020, https://olympics.nbcsports.com/2020/03/24/michael-phelps-tokyo-olympics-layden (February 27, 2022).

5. David Axelrod and Michael Phelps, "The Kennedy Forum: Michael Phelps and David Axelrod Discuss Mental Health," Kennedy Forum Illinois, January 29, 2018, YouTube video, https://youtu.be/G5mJRUur_Lk.

6. Louisa Thomas, "A Year That Changed How Athletes Think about Mental Health," *The New Yorker*, 2021, https://www.newyorker.com/culture/2021-in-review/a-year-that-changed-how-athletes-think-about-mental-health (February 27, 2022).

7. Lorenzo Reyes, "Las Vegas Raiders DC Carl Nassib: 'Has Been Good Not to Have to Lie' since Coming Out as Gay," *USA Today*, 2021, https://www.usatoday.com/story/sports/nfl/raiders/2021/08/06/carl-nassib-las-vegas-raiders-coming-out-gay/5515410001 (February 27, 2022).

8. Jonathan Chang and Meghna Chakrabarti, "How the Burden on Black Athletes Reflects the Experience of Black America," *WBUR*, 2021, https://www.wbur.org/onpoint/2021/08/04/how-the-burden-on-black-athletes-reflects-the-experience-of-black-america (February 27, 2022).

CHAPTER 1

1. Brandon Sneed, *Head in the Game* (New York: HarperCollins, 2017), 75.

2. Julie Kliegman, "Tough Breaks," *Sports Illustrated*, 2022, https://www.si.com/more-sports/2022/07/06/mental-toughness-the-strength-issue (November 6, 2022).

3. Benjamin Ide Wheeler, "A Western View of the Situation," *American Monthly Review of Reviews* 33 (1906): 72–73.

4. Jim Bauman, "The Stigma of Mental Health in Athletes: Are Mental Toughness and Mental Health Seen as Contradictory in Elite Sport?," *British Journal of Sports Medicine* 50, no. 3 (November 2015): 135–36.

5. James E. Marcia, "Ego Identity Status: Relationship to Change in Self-Esteem, 'General Maladjustment,' and Authoritarianism," *Journal of Personality* 35, no. 1 (March 1967): 118–33.

6. Alan Good, Britton Brewer, Albert Petitpas, Judy Vanraalte, and Matthew Mahar, "Identity Foreclosure, Athletic Identity, and College Sport Participation," *Academic Athletic Journal*, Spring 1993, 1–12.

7. Carmelo Anthony and D. Watkins, *Where Tomorrows Aren't Promised* (New York: Gallery Books, 2021), 57.

8. Anthony and Watkins, *Where Tomorrows Aren't Promised*, 104.

9. Sneed, *Head in the Game*, 85.

CHAPTER 2

1. Angelo Mosso, *Life of Man on the High Alps* (London: T. F. Unwin, 1898), ix.

2. Edward Wheeler Scripture, *Thinking, Feeling, Doing* (Meadville, PA: Flood and Vincent, 1895), 24.

3. Pierre de Coubertin, "La psychologie du sport," in *Olympism, Selected Writings* (Lausanne: International Olympic Committee, 2000), 146.

4. Pierre de Coubertin, "Les Congrés Olympiques," *Revue Olympique* 86 (February 1913): 19–23.

5. "Ruth Supernormal, so He Hits Homers," *New York Times*, September 11, 1921, 25(E).

6. Hugh S. Fullerton, "Why Babe Ruth Is the Greatest Home-Run Hitter," *Popular Science Monthly*, 1921, https://www.popsci.com/scitech/article/2006-10/archive-why-babe-ruth-greatest-home-run-hitter (April 30, 2022).

7. Fullerton, "Why Babe Ruth Is the Greatest Home-Run Hitter."

8. Nate Penn, "How to Build the Perfect Batter," *GQ*, September 2006, 292–305.

9. Penn, "How to Build the Perfect Batter."

10. Coleman R. Griffith, "A Laboratory for Research in Athletics," *Research Quarterly* 1, no. 3 (1930): 34–40.

11. Coleman R. Griffith, *Psychology of Coaching* (New York: Charles Scribner's Sons, 1926), 3.

12. Christopher D. Green, "Coleman Roberts Griffith: 'Father' of North American Sport Psychology," in *Psychology Gets in the Game: Sport, Mind, and Behavior, 1880–1960*, ed. Christopher D. Green and Ludy T. Benjamin (Lincoln: University of Nebraska Press, 2009), 212–13.

13. Peter Golenbock, *Wrigleyville: A Magical History Tour of the Chicago Cubs* (New York: St. Martin's Press, 1996), 272.

14. Golenbock, *Wrigleyville*, 272.

15. Paul M. Angle, *Philip K. Wrigley: A Memoir of a Modest Man* (Chicago: Rand McNally, 1975), 65.

16. Green, "Coleman Roberts Griffith," 214–16.

17. Angle, *Philip K. Wrigley*, 65.

18. Golenbock, *Wrigleyville*, 273.

19. David Farrell Tracy, *The Psychologist at Bat* (New York: Sterling Publishing, 1951), 11–16.

20. Tracy, *The Psychologist at Bat*, 16–17.

21. Tracy, *The Psychologist at Bat*, 23–26.

22. Tracy, *The Psychologist at Bat*, 29.

23. Tracy, *The Psychologist at Bat*, 30.

24. Tracy, *The Psychologist at Bat*, 29–30, 40.

25. Tracy, *The Psychologist at Bat*, 119–20.

26. Tracy, *The Psychologist at Bat*, 136.

27. Tracy, *The Psychologist at Bat*, 148–49.

28. Tracy, *The Psychologist at Bat*, 156.

29. Diane L. Gill, "History of Feminist Sport Psychology," in *Feminist Applied Sport Psychology*, ed. Leeja Carter (New York: Routledge, 2019), 21.

30. Diane L. Gill, "Women's Place in the History of Sport Psychology," *Sport Psychologist* 9 (1995): 418–33.

31. Deborah L. Feltz, "Psychosocial Perspectives on Girls and Women in Sport and Physical Activity: A Tribute to Dorothy V. Harris," *Quest* 44, no. 2 (1992): 135–37.

32. Gill, "History of Feminist Sport Psychology," 26.

33. Ruth L. Hall, "Shaking the Foundation: Women of Color in Sport," *Sport Psychologist* 15 (2001): 386–400.

34. Robert N. Singer, "Applied Sport Psychology in the United States," *Journal of Applied Sport Psychology* 1, no. 1 (1989): 61–80.

35. Green and Benjamin in *Psychology Gets in the Game*, 290.

CHAPTER 3

1. Julie Kliegman, "Paddy Steinfort and the Craft of Mental Performance Coaching," *Sports Illustrated*, 2020, https://www.si.com/edge/2020/10/02/paddy-steinfort-mental-performance-coach-daily-cover (November 12, 2022).

2. Kliegman, "Paddy Steinfort and the Craft of Mental Performance Coaching."

3. Mike Littwin, "Smoltz Escapes Losing Rut with Shrinking Pitch," *Baltimore Sun*, 1991, https://www.baltimoresun.com/news/bs-xpm-1991-10-24-1991297069-story.html (November 19, 2022).

4. Andrew Bagnato, "David Justice Endured a Bit of Ribbing," *Chicago Tribune*, 1991, https://www.chicagotribune.com/news/ct-xpm-1991-10-24-9104060078-story.html (November 22, 2022).

5. Gordon Edes, "Remembering Baseball's 'Godfather' of Mental Health Awareness: Harvey Dorfman," *Bally Sports*, 2021, https://www.ballysports.com/national/news/remembering-mlb-s-godfather-of-mental-health-awareness-harvey-dorfman (January 14, 2023).

6. Kliegman, "Paddy Steinfort and the Craft of Mental Performance Coaching."

CHAPTER 4

1. For example, on Jimmy Piersall's bipolar disorder, see Jimmy Piersall, *Fear Strikes Out* (Lincoln, NE: Bison Books, 1999).

2. Sally Jenkins, "Chamique Holdsclaw Confronts Her 'Little Secret' of Depression," *Washington Post*, 2012, https://www.washingtonpost.com/sports/othersports/chamique -holdsclaw-confronts-her-little-secret-of-depression/2012/05/17/gIQAoUe7WU_story .html (July 17, 2022).

3. Jenkins, "Chamique Holdsclaw Confronts Her 'Little Secret' of Depression."

4. "Holdsclaw Announces Retirement to a Stunned Sparks Team," *Toronto Star*, 2007, https://www.thestar.com/sports/2007/06/11/holdsclaw_announces_retirement_to _a_stunned_sparks_team.html (August 15, 2022).

5. Lauren Peterson, "Holdsclaw Explains Retirement," *Los Angeles Times*, 2007, https: //www.latimes.com/archives/la-xpm-2007-jun-21-sp-holdsclaw21-story.html (August 15, 2022).

6. Mike Tierney, "Holdsclaw Is Back in the W.N.B.A., with a Purpose," *New York Times*, 2009, https://www.nytimes.com/2009/07/11/sports/basketball/11holdsclaw.html (August 15, 2022).

7. "Holdsclaw Rebounds, Free from 'Mental Prison,'" *ESPN.com*, July 23, 2013, https://www.espn.com/womens-college-basketball/story?id=9503185&src=desk- top&rand=ref~%7B%22ref%22%3A%22 (July 19, 2022).

8. "Chamique Holdsclaw Back on Track," *Associated Press*, 2013, https://www.espn .com/espnw/news-commentary/story/_/id/9503883/chamique-holdsclaw-rebounds-free -mental-prison (July 19, 2022).

9. Buster Olney, "Harnisch Says He Is Being Treated for Depression," *New York Times*, 1997, https://www.nytimes.com/1997/04/26/sports/harnisch-says-he-is-being-treated -for-depression.html (August 14, 2022).

10. Mike Delayo, "'I Definitely Want to Thank My Psychiatrist': Digital Media Mental Health Disclosures in Professional Sports," master's thesis, Pennsylvania State University, 2021, 1.

11. Raymond I. Schuck, "'I'd Just Like to Let Everybody Know': Pete Harnisch on the Disabled List and the Politics of Mental Health," in *Sport, Rhetoric, and Political Struggle*, ed. Daniel A. Grano and Michael L. Butterworth (New York: Peter Lang, 2019), 182.

12. Robert Lipsyte, "Backtalk; Harnisch a Reluctant Role Model," *New York Times*, 1998, https://www.nytimes.com/1998/11/22/sports/backtalk-harnisch-a-reluctant-role -model.html (August 14, 2022).

13. Bill Pulsipher, "For Pulsipher, Down Doesn't Mean Out," *ESPN*, 2005, https:// www.espn.com/mlb/news/story?id=2034773 (August 4, 2022).

14. Pulsipher, "For Pulsipher, Down Doesn't Mean Out."

15. Pulsipher, "For Pulsipher, Down Doesn't Mean Out."

16. Mary Pilon, "'I'm Fucking Weird': How Royce White Became the Most Important Basketball Player Alive," *Esquire*, 2017, https://www.esquire.com/sports/a54756/royce -white-im-fucking-weird (August 8, 2022).

17. Pilon, "'I'm Fucking Weird.'"

18. Sarah Lyall, "A Player with a Cause, but without a Team," *New York Times*, 2013, https://www.nytimes.com/2013/12/10/sports/basketball/white-is-a-player-with-a-cause-but-without-a-team.html (August 9, 2022).

19. Jon Wertheim, "Royce White Takes on MMA," *Sports Illustrated*, 2020, https://www.si.com/mma/2020/04/13/royce-white-takes-on-mma (August 8, 2022).

20. Wertheim, "A Player with a Cause, but without a Team."

21. Eamon Whalen, "What Happened to Royce White?," *Mother Jones*, 2022, https://www.motherjones.com/politics/2022/08/royce-white-nba-steve-bannon-black-lives-matter (August 8, 2022).

22. Royce White, Twitter post, February 22, 2022, 10:32 a.m., https://twitter.com/Highway_30/status/1496145597056880649.

23. David Gardner, "How a Former NBA Player and Activist Became a Far-Right Media Darling," *Washington Post*, 2022, https://www.washingtonpost.com/sports/2022/04/28/royce-white-nba-minnesota-congress/ (August 14, 2022).

24. Royce White, "An Open Letter to the Democrats," *The Official Substack of Royce White*, 2022, https://roycewhite.substack.com/p/an-open-letter-to-the-democrats (August 9, 2022).

25. Sean Gregory, "Why Activist Royce White Thinks NBA Players Should Get Out of the Bubble and Onto the Street," *Time*, 2020, https://time.com/5884598/royce-white-nba-minneapolis-protests (August 9, 2022).

26. Whalen, "What Happened to Royce White?"

27. Julie Kliegman, "The State of Mental Health Care in the NBA," *The Ringer*, 2018, https://www.theringer.com/nba/2018/5/7/17320362/mental-health-nba (August 8, 2022).

28. Susan Scutti, "Michael Phelps: 'I Am Extremely Thankful That I Did Not Take My Life,'" *CNN*, 2018, https://www.cnn.com/2018/01/19/health/michael-phelps-depression (July 30, 2022).

29. Tim Layden, "After Rehabilitation, the Best of Michael Phelps May Lie Ahead," *Sports Illustrated*, 2015, https://www.si.com/olympics/2015/11/09/michael-phelps-rehabilitation-rio-2016 (July 30, 2022)

30. Layden, "After Rehabilitation, the Best of Michael Phelps May Lie Ahead."

31. Julie Kliegman, "Michael Phelps on Mental Health and the USOPC: 'I Want People to Actually Do Something,'" *Sports Illustrated*, 2022, https://www.si.com/olympics/2022/10/10/michael-phelps-mental-health-advocacy-sports-nft-cover (December 10, 2022).

32. Kliegman, "After Rehabilitation, the Best of Michael Phelps May Lie Ahead."

33. Scutti, "Michael Phelps."

34. Matthew Futterman, "Michael Phelps: 'I Can't See Any More Suicides,'" *New York Times*, 2020, https://www.nytimes.com/2020/07/29/sports/olympics/michael-phelps-documentary-weight-of-gold.html (July 30, 2022).

35. Andy Bull, "The Life and Death of Steve Holcomb, Forever Seeking That Perfect Line," *The Guardian*, 2018, https://www.theguardian.com/sport/2018/feb/06/steve-holcomb-blind-bobsled-winter-olympics (August 2, 2022).

36. Johnny Brayson, "Steven Holcomb's Appearance in 'The Weight of Gold' Is a Reminder of an Olympian Gone Too Soon," *Bustle*, 2020, https://www.bustle.com/entertainment/steven-holcomb-appearance-hbo-weight-of-gold (August 2, 2022).

37. Kliegman, "After Rehabilitation, the Best of Michael Phelps May Lie Ahead."

CHAPTER 5

1. DeMar DeRozan, Twitter post, February 17, 2018, 6:06 a.m., https://twitter.com/demar_derozan/status/964818383303688197?lang=en.

2. Doug Smith, "Raptors' DeMar DeRozan Hopes Honest Talk on Depression Helps Others," *Toronto Star*, 2018, https://www.thestar.com/sports/raptors/2018/02/25/raptors-derozan-hopes-honest-talk-on-depression-helps-others.html (October 2, 2022).

3. Smith, "Raptors' DeMar DeRozan Hopes Honest Talk on Depression Helps Others."

4. "VanVleet: DeRozan Changed NBA by 'Speaking Out' about Mental Health," *Sportsnet*, 2020, https://www.sportsnet.ca/nba/article/vanvleet-derozan-changed-nba-speaking-mental-health (October 16, 2022).

5. Kevin Love, "Everyone Is Going through Something," *Players' Tribune*, 2018, https://www.theplayerstribune.com/articles/kevin-love-everyone-is-going-through-something (October 2, 2022).

6. Love, "Everyone Is Going through Something."

7. Love, "Everyone Is Going through Something."

8. Love, "Everyone Is Going through Something."

9. DeMar DeRozan, Twitter post, March 7, 2018, 11:45 a.m., https://twitter.com/DeMar_DeRozan/status/971426505128644614.

10. "DeMar DeRozan on Inspiring Kevin Love: 'Made Me Feel Pretty Damn Good,'" *ESPN*, 2018, https://www.espn.com/nba/story/_/id/22672925/demar-derozan-grateful-inspired-kevin-love-discuss-mental-health (October 8, 2022).

11. A. J. Neuharth-Keusch, "DeMar DeRozan Proud to Have Been 'Sacrificial Lamb' for Kevin Love, Others," *USA Today*, 2018, https://www.usatoday.com/story/sports/nba/2018/03/07/demar-derozan-proud-kevin-love-others-mental-health/402634002 (October 8, 2022).

12. Michael Lee, "How the NBA Got Serious about Mental Health," *Washington Post*, 2022, https://www.washingtonpost.com/sports/2022/04/19/nba-mental-health-demar-derozan (October 15, 2022).

13. "Kelly Oubre, Jr. Goes 1-on-1 to Talk Depression, Anxiety, and Mental Health," *Wizards Talk*, 2018, https://art19.com/shows/wizards-tipoff/episodes/f5437f70-b77e-40b3-860a-65b0dbf923a9 (October 8, 2022).

14. David MacKay, "Steve Kerr Voices Appreciation for Kevin Love Discussing Mental Health," *USA Today*, 2018, https://warriorswire.usatoday.com/2018/03/06/steve-kerr-kevin-love-mental-health (October 11, 2022).

15. LeBron James, Twitter post, March 6, 2018, 11:01 a.m., https://twitter.com/KingJames/status/971053228950544384.

16. Robin Lehner, "'I Could Not Stand Being Alone in My Brain': Islanders Goalie Robin Lehner Opens Up about His Addiction and Bipolar Diagnosis," *The Athletic*,

2018, https://theathletic.com/522117/2018/09/13/islanders-goalie-robin-lehner-opens-up-about-his-addiction-and-bipolar-diagnosis-i-could-not-stand-being-alone-in-my-brain (October 11, 2022).

17. Anne Branigin, "WNBA Star Skylar Diggins, Fed Up with Lack of Support, Reveals She Played Entire 2018 Season while Pregnant," *The Root*, 2019, https://www.theroot.com/wnba-star-skylar-diggins-fed-up-with-lack-of-support-1839232084 (October 11, 2022).

18. Claire Gillespie, "Serena Williams Explains Why She Doesn't Use the Term 'Postpartum Depression,'" *Self*, 2018, https://www.self.com/story/serena-williams-doesnt-use-the-term-postpartum-depression (October 11, 2022).

19. Mike Delayo, "'I Definitely Want to Thank My Psychiatrist': Digital Media Mental Health Disclosures in Professional Sports," master's thesis, Pennsylvania State University, 2021, 79.

20. Larry Sanders, "Why I Walked Away from the NBA," *Players' Tribune*, 2015, https://www.theplayerstribune.com/articles/larry-sanders-exclusive-interview (October 22, 2022).

21. Mirin Fader, "The Many Dimensions of DeMar DeRozan," *The Ringer*, 2022, https://www.theringer.com/nba/2022/2/18/22939702/demar-derozan-chicago-bulls-all-star (October 16, 2022).

22. Liz Cambage, "DNP-Mental Health," *Players' Tribune*, 2019, https://www.theplayerstribune.com/articles/liz-cambage-mental-health (October 15, 2022).

23. Cambage, "DNP-Mental Health."

24. Delayo, "'I Definitely Want to Thank My Psychiatrist,'" 43.

25. Jackie Powell, "The WNBA Is Finally Catching Up on Mental Health," *Sports Illustrated*, 2021, https://www.si.com/wnba/2021/08/19/mental-health-illness-wnbpa-speaking-out (October 15, 2022).

26. Powell, "The WNBA Is Finally Catching Up on Mental Health."

27. Corey Hirsch, "Dark, Dark, Dark, Dark, Dark, Dark, Dark, Dark," *Players' Tribune*, 2017, https://www.theplayerstribune.com/articles/corey-hirsch-dark-dark-dark (October 16, 2022).

28. Nicole Yang, "At Sloan, NBA Commissioner Adam Silver Talks Candidly about Players' Mental Health," *Boston.com*, 2019, https://www.boston.com/sports/nba/2019/03/01/adam-silver-sloan-nba-unhappy (October 23, 2022).

29. Melissa Yang, "Soccer Star Christen Press Is Done Suffering for Success," *GQ*, 2022, https://www.gq.com/story/christen-press-interview-angel-city-football-club (October 23, 2022).

CHAPTER 6

1. "U.S. Open, September 2, 2019," *ASAP Sports*, 2019, http://www.asapsports.com/show_interview.php?id=153355 (November 23, 2022).

2. Jill Martin, "Naomi Osaka Says She Won't Do Press Conferences at the French Open," *CNN*, 2021, https://www.cnn.com/2021/05/26/tennis/naomi-osaka-no-press-conferences-at-french-open-spt-intl/index.html (April 12, 2021).

3. Ryan Wilson, "Report: Marshawn Lynch Trademarks 'I'm Just Here so I Won't Get Fined,'" *CBS Sports*, 2015, https://www.cbssports.com/nfl/news/report-marshawn-lynch -trademarks-im-just-here-so-i-wont-get-fined (April 12, 2022).

4. Krystie Lee Yandoli, "Naomi Osaka Said She Won't Do News Conferences at the French Open to Protect Her Mental Health," *BuzzFeed News*, 2021, https:// www.buzzfeednews.com/article/krystieyandoli/naomi-osaka-news-conferences-mental -health (November 26, 2022).

5. D'Arcy Maine, "Naomi Osaka to Skip News Conferences at French Open, Citing Importance of Mental Health," *ESPN*, 2021, https://www.espn.com/tennis/story/ _/id/31517078/naomi-osaka-skip-news-conferences-french-open-citing-mental-health (November 26, 2022).

6. Billie Jean King, Twitter post, May 30, 2021, 6:01 p.m., https://twitter.com/ BillieJeanKing/status/1399123726239666176.

7. Liz Clarke, "Naomi Osaka Fined $15,000 for Skipping French Open News Conference; Grand Slams Issue Warning," *Washington Post*, 2021, https://www.washingtonpost .com/sports/2021/05/30/naomi-osaka-french-open-fine (November 27, 2022).

8. Piers Morgan, "Narcissistic Naomi's Cynical Exploitation of Mental Health to Silence the Media Is Right from the Meghan and Harry Playbook of Wanting Their Press Cake and Eating It," *Daily Mail*, 2021, https://www.dailymail.co.uk/news/article -9636993/PIERS-MORGAN-Narcissistic-Naomis-cynical-exploitation-mental-health -silence-media.html (November 27, 2022).

9. Tumaini Carayol, "Naomi Osaka Fined for Media Snub and Threatened with French Open Expulsion," *The Guardian*, 2021, https://www.theguardian.com/sport/2021/may/30 /french-open-womens-singles-naomi-osaka-patricia-tig (May 9, 2022).

10. Naomi Osaka, Instagram post, May 30, 2021, https://www.instagram.com/p/ CPi9kJHJfxO.

11. Billie Jean King, Twitter post, May 31, 2021, 4:19 p.m., https://twitter.com/ billiejeanking/status/1399460549407219712?lang=en.

12. Alex Abad-Santos, "Naomi Osaka and Tennis Journalism's Ugly History of Demeaning Its Players," *Vox*, 2021, https://www.vox.com/22534957/naomi-osaka-french -open-wimbledon (November 27, 2022).

13. Morgan Jerkins, "Naomi Osaka's Next Chapter," *Self*, 2022, https://www.self.com/ story/naomi-osaka (May 9, 2022).

14. Simone Biles, Twitter post, January 15, 2018, 4:22 p.m., https://twitter.com/ Simone_Biles/status/953014513837715457.

15. Devlin Barrett, "Simone Biles to Congress: 'I Blame Larry Nassar, and I Also Blame an Entire System,'" *Washington Post*, 2021, https://www.washingtonpost.com /national-security/gymnasts-nassar-fbi-investigation-hearing/2021/09/14/de4832cc -159f-11ec-9589-31ac3173c2e5_story.html (April 24, 2022).

16. Camonghne Felix, "Simone Biles Chose Herself," *The Cut*, 2021, https://www .thecut.com/article/simone-biles-olympics-2021.html (May 1, 2022).

17. Mike Gavin, "Simone Biles Opens Up about Twisties, Olympics Timeline, and Experience," *NBC Philadelphia*, 2021, https://www.nbcphiladelphia.com/news/

sports/tokyo-summer-olympics/simone-biles-opens-up-about-twisties-tokyo-olympics
-timeline-and-experience/2912546 (April 24, 2022).

18. George Ramsay, John Sinnott, and Rebecca Wright, "'I Have to Focus on My Mental Health,' Says Simone Biles after Withdrawing from Gold Medal Event," *CNN*, 2021, https://www.cnn.com/2021/07/27/sport/simone-biles-tokyo-2020-olympics/index.html (April 24, 2022).

19. Simone Biles, Twitter post, July 28, 2021, 9:46 p.m., https://twitter.com/simone
_biles/status/1420561448883802118.

20. Dan Wetzel, "Simone Biles: 'I Didn't Quit . . . My Mind and Body Are Simply Not in Sync,'" *Yahoo* 2021, https://sports.yahoo.com/simone-biles-i-didnt-quit-my-mind
-body-are-simply-not-in-sync-060622826.html?guccounter=1 (May 1, 2022).

21. Stephanie Apstein, "Former Gymnasts Left Paralyzed Are No Stranger to the Struggles Biles Faced," *Sports Illustrated*, 2021, https://www.si.com/olympics/2021/08
/02/simone-biles-twisties-physical-risk-former-gymnasts-left-paralyzed (May 1, 2022).

22. Felix, "Simone Biles Chose Herself."

23. Merrit Kennedy and Leila Fadel, "She's Still Dealing with the Twisties, but Simone Biles Wins Another Medal in Tokyo," *NPR*, 2021, https://www.npr.org/sections/tokyo
-olympics-live-updates/2021/08/03/1024122723/simone-biles-return-balance-beam
-gymnastics-olympics (November 27, 2022).

24. Maura Hohman, "Simone Biles Says Winning Bronze on Beam 'Means More Than All the Golds,'" *Today*, 2021, https://www.today.com/news/simone-biles-reflects
-winning-bronze-beam-today-t227184 (May 1, 2022).

25. Jason Campbell, Twitter post, July 27, 2021, 4:44 p.m., https://twitter.com/
JasonSCampbell/status/1420122875323985920.

26. Wil Leitner, "Why You Shouldn't Praise Simone Biles for Quitting Tokyo Olympics," *The Ben Maller Show*, 2021, https://foxsportsradio.iheart.com/featured/the-ben
-maller-show/content/2021-07-29-why-you-shouldnt-praise-simone-biles-for-quitting
-tokyo-olympics (May 1, 2022).

27. Matt Young, "Texas Deputy Attorney General Aaron Reitz Calls Simone Biles an 'Embarrassment,'" *Chron*, 2021, https://www.chron.com/sports/article/Texas-attorney
-general-Aaron-Reitz-Simone-Biles-16345527.php (November 27, 2022).

28. Jemele Hill, "Simone Biles's Critics Don't Understand This Generation of Athletes," *The Atlantic*, 2021, https://www.theatlantic.com/ideas/archive/2021/07/simone
-biles-doesnt-need-to-look-invincible/619606 (May 1, 2022).

29. Zac Al-Khateeb, "Michael Phelps Gives Impassioned Defense of Simone Biles' Mental Health: 'It's OK to Not Be OK,'" *Sporting News*, 2021, https://www
.sportingnews.com/us/athletics/news/michael-phelps-simone-biles-mental-health/
ja1pgywo7t1y1qv0un5g39l2a (May 1, 2022).

30. Adam Rippon, Twitter post, July 27, 2021, 9:21 a.m., https://twitter.com/
AdamRippon/status/1420011455152275457.

31. "AOC Says Simone Biles Taking Her Olympic Break Was Good on All Fronts," *TMZ*, 2021, https://www.tmz.com/2021/08/03/alexandria-ocasio-cortez-aoc-simone
-biles-mental-health-olympics (May 1, 2022).

32. Justin Bieber, Instagram post, July 28, 2021, https://www.instagram.com/p/CR4b2HrHBrT.

33. Katie Kindelan, "Simone Biles Ties Mental Health Struggle at Tokyo Olympics to Nassar Sexual Abuse," *Good Morning America*, 2021, https://www.goodmorningamerica.com/wellness/story/simone-biles-ties-mental-health-struggle-tokyo-olympics-80038932 (December 29, 2022).

34. Bianca Andreescu, Twitter post, December 6, 2021, 12:04 p.m., https://twitter.com/Bandreescu_/status/1467902871442239499.

35. Julie Kliegman, "Michael Phelps on Mental Health and the USOPC: 'I Want People to Actually Do Something,'" *Sports Illustrated*, 2022, https://www.si.com/olympics/2022/10/10/michael-phelps-mental-health-advocacy-sports-nft-cover (November 27, 2022).

36. Naomi Osaka, "Naomi Osaka: It's O.K. to Not Be O.K.," *Time*, 2021, https://time.com/6077128/naomi-osaka-essay-tokyo-olympics (May 5, 2022).

37. D'Arcy Maine, "Naomi Osaka Addresses Crowd after Fan Heckles Her during Loss at Indian Wells," *ESPN*, 2022, https://www.espn.com/tennis/story/_/id/33490935/naomi-osaka-addresses-crowd-fan-heckles-loss-indian-wells (May 5, 2022).

38. L. Jon Wertheim, "We Should Put Naomi Osaka's Well-Being First, Not Take Sides in a Mental Health Debate," *Sports Illustrated*, 2022, https://www.si.com/tennis/2022/03/14/naomi-osaka-indian-wells-heckled-by-fan-questions (May 5, 2022).

CHAPTER 7

1. Scott Hanson, "Former WSU Star Receiver Gabe Marks Wants to Help Football Players with Their Mental Health," *Seattle Times*, 2022, https://www.seattletimes.com/sports/wsu-cougars/former-wsu-star-receiver-gabe-marks-wants-to-help-football-players-with-their-mental-health (May 29, 2022).

2. Julie Kliegman, "College Athletes Are Only Starting to Get Access to the Mental Health Care They Need," *The Ringer*, 2017, https://www.theringer.com/2017/10/26/16535274/ncaa-student-athletes-mental-health-care-initiatives (May 13, 2022).

3. Kliegman, "College Athletes Are Only Starting to Get Access to the Mental Health Care They Need."

4. Kate Fagan, "Split Image," *ESPN*, 2015, http://www.espn.com/espn/feature/story/_/id/12833146/instagram-account-university-pennsylvania-runner-showed-only-part-story (May 28, 2022).

5. Julie Kliegman, "Sarah Fuller's Journey from Football Kicker to Mental Health Advocate," *Sports Illustrated*, 2022, https://www.si.com/college/2022/07/25/sarah-fuller-vanderbilt-football-daily-cover (October 30, 2022).

6. Scott Stump, "Parents of Stanford Soccer Team Captain Katie Meyer Speak Out about Her Death," *Today*, 2022, https://www.today.com/news/sports/katie-meyer-death-parents-interview-rcna18694 (May 23, 2022).

7. Jenni Carlson, "How JMU Catcher Lauren Bernett's Death Rocked College Softball and Pushed It to Action on Mental Health," *USA Today*, 2022, https://www.usatoday.com/story/sports/college/softball/2022/05/09/lauren-bernett-suicide-jmu-college-softball-world-mental-health/9703602002 (May 24, 2022).

8. "Who We Are," Dam Worth It Co., https://www.damworthit.co/our-mission (June 13, 2022).

CHAPTER 8

1. Julie Kliegman, "What Do Athletes Get from Ayahuasca, Mushrooms, and Ecstasy?" *Sports Illustrated*, 2022, https://www.si.com/more-sports/2022/08/12/psychedelics-sports -aaron-rodgers-daily-cover (December 25, 2022).

2. Briana Scurry, with Wayne Coffey, *My Greatest Save: The Brave, Barrier-Breaking Journey of a World Champion Goalkeeper* (New York: Abrams Press, 2022), 7.

3. Drew Weisholtz, "TODAY Exclusive: Sha'Carri Richardson Speaks Out about Failing Drug Test Ahead of Olympics," *Today*, 2021, https://www.today.com/news/ today-show-exclusive-sha-carri-richardson-speaks-out-about-failing-t224363 (December 24, 2022).

4. Julie Kliegman, "Michael Phelps on Mental Health and the USOPC: 'I Want People to Actually Do Something,'" *Sports Illustrated*, 2022, https://www.si.com/olympics/2022 /10/10/michael-phelps-mental-health-advocacy-sports-nft-cover (December 11, 2022).

5. CC Sabathia and Chris Smith, *Till the End* (New York: Random House, 2021), 71.

6. Sabathia and Smith, *Till the End*, 161.

7. Sabathia and Smith, *Till the End*, 195.

8. Sabathia and Smith, *Till the End*, 217.

9. Sabathia and Smith, *Till the End*, 221.

10. "CC Sabathia Explains His Decision to Enter Rehab," *Good Morning America*, 2015, https://www.goodmorningamerica.com/news/video/cc-sabathia-explains-decision -enter-rehab-34998129 (December 11, 2022).

11. Bob Welch and George Vecsey, *Five O'Clock Comes Early: A Young Man's Battle with Alcoholism* (Indianapolis: Quill, 1981), 14.

12. Welch and Vecsey, *Five O'Clock Comes Early*, 44–45.

13. Sabathia and Smith, *Till the End*, 229.

14. Kliegman, "What Do Athletes Get from Ayahuasca, Mushrooms, and Ecstasy?"

15. Kliegman, "What Do Athletes Get from Ayahuasca, Mushrooms, and Ecstasy?"

16. Kliegman, "What Do Athletes Get from Ayahuasca, Mushrooms, and Ecstasy?"

17. Aubrey Marcus, "Aaron Rodgers' Challenging Journey to Self Love and Mental Health," *YouTube*, 2022, https://www.youtube.com/watch?v=Px3_lDaXHJM (December 25, 2022).

18. Kliegman, "What Do Athletes Get from Ayahuasca, Mushrooms, and Ecstasy?"

19. Kliegman, "What Do Athletes Get from Ayahuasca, Mushrooms, and Ecstasy?"

CHAPTER 9

1. Kate Bennett, *Treating Athletes with Eating Disorders* (New York: Routledge, 2022), 31.

2. Mary Cain, "I Was the Fastest Girl in America, until I Joined Nike," *New York Times*, 2019, https://www.nytimes.com/2019/11/07/opinion/nike-running-mary-cain .html (April 10, 2022).

3. Cain, "I Was the Fastest Girl in America, until I Joined Nike."

4. Maggie Astor, "A Gymnast's Death Was Supposed to Be a Wake-Up Call. What Took So Long?," *New York Times*, 2022, https://www.nytimes.com/2022/04/26/sports/christy-henrich-gymnastics-eating-disorder-death.html (May 29, 2022).

5. Monica Seles, *Getting a Grip: On My Body, My Mind, My Self* (New York: Avery, 2009), 97, 104, 108.

6. Seles, *Getting a Grip*, 103, 110, 116, 118.

7. Seles, *Getting a Grip*, 2.

8. Bennett, *Treating Athletes with Eating Disorders*, 3–4.

CHAPTER 10

1. Julie Kliegman, "Mentally, That's a Whole 'Nother Ball Game," *Sports Illustrated*, 2020, https://www.si.com/olympics/2020/04/29/mental-impact-of-the-pandemic-on-athletes (July 25, 2022).

2. Kliegman, "Mentally, That's a Whole 'Nother Ball Game."

3. Laurie Tarkan, "Athletes' Injuries Go beyond the Physical," *New York Times*, 2000, https://www.nytimes.com/2000/09/26/health/athletes-injuries-go-beyond-the-physical.html (July 25, 2022).

4. Diane M. Wiese-Bjornstal, Aynsley M. Smith, Shelly M. Shaffer, and Michael A. Morrey, "An Integrated Model of Response to Sport Injury: Psychological and Sociological Dynamics," *Journal of Applied Sport Psychology* 10, no. 1 (1998): 46–69.

5. Percy Allen, "Despite Challenges of Rehab, Storm Star Breanna Stewart Thinks She Can Be Better Than Ever," *Seattle Times*, 2019, https://www.seattletimes.com/sports/storm/i-can-be-better-than-what-i-was-despite-challenges-of-rehab-storm-star-breanna-stewart-is-confident-in-her-comeback (July 26, 2022).

6. Douglas Robson, "Serena Williams Depressed but Determined to Return to Top," *USA Today*, 2011, https://usatoday30.usatoday.com/sports/tennis/2011-03-15-serena-williams-interview_N.htm (July 27, 2022).

7. Hannah Webster, "How to Overcome Depression after a Sports Injury," *Yahoo!*, 2014, https://news.yahoo.com/overcome-depression-sports-injury-155401670.html (July 27, 2022).

8. Kliegman, "Mentally, That's a Whole 'Nother Ball Game."

9. Kliegman, "Mentally, That's a Whole 'Nother Ball Game."

10. Kliegman, "Mentally, That's a Whole 'Nother Ball Game."

11. Kliegman, "Mentally, That's a Whole 'Nother Ball Game."

12. Kliegman, "Mentally, That's a Whole 'Nother Ball Game."

13. Edwin Rosenberg, "Athletic Retirement as Social Death: Concepts and Perspectives," in *Sport and the Sociological Imagination*, ed. Nancy Theberge and Peter Donnelly (Fort Worth: Texas Christian University Press, 1982), 246.

14. Briana Scurry and Wayne Coffey, *My Greatest Save: The Brave, Barrier-Breaking Journey of a World Champion Goalkeeper* (New York: Abrams Press, 2022), 197.

15. Bill Bradley, *Life on the Run* (New York: Bantam Books, 1976), 191.

16. Jim Bouton, *Ball Four* (New York: Dell, 1970), 56.

17. Rosenberg, "Athletic Retirement as Social Death," 246.

18. Kliegman, "Mentally, That's a Whole 'Nother Ball Game."

CONCLUSION

1. Briana Scurry and Wayne Coffey, *My Greatest Save: The Brave, Barrier-Breaking Journey of a World Champion Goalkeeper* (New York: Abrams Press, 2022), 230.

2. "Heat's Erik Spoelstra Believes Mental Health Will Become Main Topic among Coaches in Offseason," *Palm Beach Post*, 2018, https://www.palmbeachpost.com/story/sports/nba/2018/03/20/heat-s-erik-spoelstra-believes/6881630007 (January 6, 2023).

3. Joanne P. McCallie, *Secret Warrior: A Coach and Fighter, On and Off the Court* (Virginia Beach, VA: Koehler Books, 2021), 64.

4. Julie Kliegman, "'I Wasn't Really Doing It for Myself,'" *Sports Illustrated*, 2023, https://www.si.com/nba/2023/01/24/tyrell-terry-nba-stanford-retire-mental-health-daily-cover (February 4, 2023).

5. Kliegman, "'I Wasn't Really Doing It for Myself.'"

SELECT BIBLIOGRAPHY

Note: This bibliography includes all sources not cited in the endnotes as well as those materials used extensively in the research of this work.

"A Brief History of Tennis." *International Olympic Committee*. 2017. https://olympics.com/ioc/news/a-brief-history-of-tennis (March 5, 2022).

Adhia, Avanti, Alice M. Ellyson, and Emily Kroshus. "Prevalence and Formal Reporting of Sexual Violence among Undergraduate Student-Athletes: A Multi-State Study." *Journal of Interpersonal Violence* 38, no. 1–2 (April 2022): 418–42.

AlBaroudi, Wajih. "Sharon Robinson Shares Essayist's Emotional Story." *MLB*. 2019. https://www.mlb.com/news/sharon-robinson-rbi-world-series (October 30, 2022).

Anshel, Mark H. *APA Handbook of Sport and Exercise Psychology*. Vol. 1. Washington, DC: American Psychological Association, 2019.

Anthony, Carmelo, and D. Watkins. *Where Tomorrows Aren't Promised*. New York: Gallery Books, 2021.

Apstein, Stephanie. "How Simone Biles Came Back to Win the Bronze of Her Life." *Sports Illustrated*. 2021. https://www.si.com/olympics/2021/08/03/simone-biles-bronze-beam-tokyo-olympics-comeback-daily-cover (May 4, 2022).

Arnold, Chris. "Naomi Osaka Drops Out of French Open after Dispute over Media Appearances." *NPR*. 2021. https://www.npr.org/2021/05/31/1001917952/naomi-osaka-drops-out-of-french-open-after-dispute-over-media-appearances (April 12, 2022).

Ayton, Agnes, and Ali Ibrahim. "Does UK Medical Education Provide Doctors with Sufficient Skills and Knowledge to Manage Patients with Eating Disorders Safely?" *Postgraduate Medical Journal* 94, no. 3 (June 2018): 374–80.

Beamon, Krystal. "'I'm a Baller': Athletic Identity Foreclosure among African American Former Student-Athletes." *Journal of African American Studies* 16 (June 2012): 195–208.

Beard, Amanda, and Rebecca Paley. *In the Water They Can't See You Cry: A Memoir*. New York: Gallery Books, 2013.

Bennett, Kate. *Treating Athletes with Eating Disorders: Bridging the Gap between Sport and Clinical Worlds*. New York: Routledge, 2022.

Boren, Cindy. "Lane Johnson, Calvin Ridley Show Mental Health Is Becoming Less of a Taboo Topic in the NFL." *Washington Post*. 2021. https://www.washingtonpost.com/sports/2021/11/01/nfl-mental-health-calvin-ridley-lane-johnson (February 10, 2023).

Brown, Gary T., ed. "Mind, Body and Sport." *NCAA*. 2014. http://www.ncaapublications.com/productdownloads/MindBodySport.pdf (July 25, 2022).

Browne, Grace. "The Therapy Part of Psychedelic Therapy Is a Mess." *Wired*. 2023. https://www.wired.com/story/psychedelic-therapy-mess (April 20, 2023).

Campbell, Ken. "More Explosive and Shocking Allegations against Junior Hockey in Newly Filed Lawsuit." *Hockey News*. 2020. https://thehockeynews.com/news/more-explosive-and-shocking-allegations-against-junior-hockey-in-newly-filed-lawsuit (December 10, 2022).

Carayol, Tumaini. "Naomi Osaka Withdraws from French Open amid Row over Press Conferences." *Guardian*. 2021. https://www.theguardian.com/sport/2021/may/31/naomi-osaka-withdraws-french-open-press-conference-fines-tennis (November 26, 2022).

Carpenter, Les. "Nearly Two Years after a Life-Threatening Injury, Alex Smith Completes an Impossible Comeback." *Washington Post*. 2020. https://www.washingtonpost.com/sports/nearly-two-years-after-a-life-threatening-injury-alex-smith-completes-an-impossible-comeback/2020/10/11/d772c99a-0be0-11eb-8074-0e943a91bf08_story.html (July 26, 2022).

Carter, Leeja, ed. *Feminist Applied Sport Psychology: From Theory to Practice*. New York: Routledge, 2019.

Cha, Boseok, Jeong Hyun Kim, Tae Hyon Ha, Jae Seung Chang, and Kyooseob Ha. "Polarity of the First Episode and Time to Diagnosis of Bipolar I Disorder." *Psychiatry Investigation* 6, no. 2 (June 2009): 96–101.

Champlin, Reid. "When College Students Want Mental Health Help but Get Stuck Waiting in Line." *Vice*. 2019. https://www.vice.com/en/article/evjqwz/college-mental-health-center-wait-times (May 24, 2022).

Chen, Anelise. *So Many Olympic Exertions*. Los Angeles: Kaya Press, 2017.

Clemmons, Anna Katherine. "Pushed by Players, the N.F.L. Works to Embrace Mental Health." *New York Times*. 2021. https://www.nytimes.com/2021/11/26/sports/football/nfl-mental-health.html (February 10, 2023).

———. "'No One Is Shying Away from That Conversation.'" *New York Times*. 2022. https://www.nytimes.com/2022/09/30/sports/football/indianapolis-colts-mental-health.html (February 13, 2023).

"College Football and Its Civil War Symbols." *Atlanta Journal-Constitution*. 2017. https://www.ajc.com/sports/college/college-football-and-its-civil-war-symbols/IvLS6thfJBcWhMXGTqWx5N (March 5, 2022).

Conviser, Jenny, Sheehan D. Fisher, and Susanna A. McColley. "Are Children with Chronic Illnesses Requiring Dietary Therapy at Risk for Disordered Eating or Eating Disorders? A Systematic Review." *International Journal of Eating Disorders* 51, no. 3 (March 2018): 187–213.

Crouse, Karen. "Gracie Gold's Battle for Olympic Glory Ended in a Fight to Save Herself." *New York Times*. 2019. https://www.nytimes.com/2019/01/25/sports/gracie-gold-figure-skating-.html (February 26, 2023).

Davidson, Neil. "Canadian Goalkeeper Stephanie Labbé Opens Up about Mental Health Struggles during Tokyo Olympics." 2021. https://www.cbc.ca/sports/soccer/stephanie-labb%C3%A9-opens-up-about-mental-health-struggles-during-olympics-1.6186844 (February 10, 2023).

Delayo, Mike. "'I Definitely Want to Thank My Psychiatrist': Digital Media Mental Health Disclosures in Professional Sports." Master's thesis, Pennsylvania State University. 2021.

Dewsbury, Donald A., Ludy T. Benjamin Jr., and Michael Wertheimer. *Portraits of Pioneers in Psychology*. Vol. 6. Washington, DC: American Psychological Association and Lawrence Erlbaum Associates, 2006.

Dinich, Heather. "Maryland Agrees to Settle with Family of Jordan McNair for $3.5 Million." *ESPN*. 2021. https://www.espn.com/college-football/story/_/id/30719018/maryland-agrees-settle-family-jordan-mcnair-35-million (March 5, 2022).

Dorfman, Harvey A. *Coaching the Mental Game: Leadership Philosophies and Strategies for Peak Performance in Sports—and Everyday Life*. Lanham, MD: Taylor Trade Publishing, 2003.

Elbaba, Julia. "How NCAA Transfer Portal Works and What It Means for Players." *NBC Sports Washington*. 2022. https://www.nbcsports.com/washington/ncaa/how-ncaa-transfer-portal-works-and-what-it-means-players (October 30, 2022).

Fagan, Kate. *The Reappearing Act: Coming Out as Gay on a College Basketball Team Led by Born-Again Christians*. New York: Skyhorse, 2014.

———. *What Made Maddy Run: The Secret Struggles and Tragic Death of an All-American Teen*. Boston: Little, Brown, 2017.

Farber, Michael. "Labbé: A Story of Depression, a Bronze Medal and the Power of Resilience." *Team Canada*. 2019. https://olympic.ca/2019/01/28/labbe-a-story-of-depression-a-bronze-medal-and-the-power-of-resilience (May 3, 2022).

Felix, Camonghne. "Simone Biles Chose Herself." *The Cut*. 2021. https://www.thecut.com/article/simone-biles-olympics-2021.html (May 1, 2022).

Fickman, Laurie. "Have the Conversation: Mental Health Expert Says Suicide Prevention Starts with Talking." *University of Houston*. 2022. https://www.uh.edu/news-events/stories/sept.-2022/09012022-suicide-prevention-month-walker.php (December 4, 2022).

"The First Game: November 6, 1869." *Rutgers University Athletics*. https://scarletknights.com/sports/2022/7/25/sports-m-footbl-archive-first-game-html.aspx (March 5, 2022).

Fullerton, Hugh S. "Why Babe Ruth Is the Greatest Home-Run Hitter." *Popular Science Monthly*. 1921. https://www.popsci.com/scitech/article/2006-10/archive-why-babe-ruth-greatest-home-run-hitter (April 30, 2022).

Futterman, Matthew. "Naomi Osaka Says She Won't Talk to Journalists at the French Open." *New York Times*. 2021. https://www.nytimes.com/2021/05/26/sports/tennis/naomi-osaka-french-open-no-interviews.html (April 12, 2022).

Ganguli, Tania. "How Some Lakers Are Using Meditation to Elevate Their Game." *Los Angeles Times*. 2018. https://www.latimes.com/sports/lakers/la-sp-lakers-meditation-20181217-story.html (February 27, 2022).

Gardner, Frank, and Zella Moore. *Clinical Sport Psychology*. Champaign, IL: Human Kinetics, 2005.

Giambalvo, Emily. "Simone Biles Said She Got the 'Twisties.' Gymnasts Immediately Understood." *Washington Post*. 2021. https://www.washingtonpost.com/sports/olympics/2021/07/28/twisties-gymnastics-simone-biles-tokyo-olympics (May 1, 2022).

Ginsburg, David. "Maryland Takes Responsibility for Mistakes in Player Death." *Associated Press*. 2018. https://apnews.com/article/84f32c339ae8496784b3e174d94f7da3 (March 5, 2022).

Goldich, Mitch. "Simone Biles Reveals Details on 'Twisties' Problem." *Sports Illustrated*. 2021. https://www.si.com/olympics/2021/07/30/simone-biles-explains-twisties-problem-details-instagram (May 1, 2022).

Gorman, Kimberly S. "Annual Survey." *Association for University and College Counseling Center Directors*. 2020. https://www.aucccd.org/assets/documents/Survey/2019-2020%20Annual%20Report%20FINAL%20March-2021.pdf (May 24, 2022).

Grano, Daniel L., and Michael Butterworth, eds. *Sport, Rhetoric, and Political Struggle*. New York: Peter Lang, 2019.

Green, Christopher D. "Psychology Strikes Out: Coleman R. Griffith and the Chicago Cubs." *History of Psychology* 6, no. 3 (August 2003): 267–83.

Green, Christopher D., and Ludy T. Benjamin, eds. *Psychology Gets in the Game: Sport, Mind, and Behavior, 1880–1960*. Lincoln: University of Nebraska Press, 2009.

Greenberg, Doug. "Paige Bueckers Adds Crocs to Impressive List of NIL Sponsors." *Front Office Sports*. 2022. https://frontofficesports.com/paige-bueckers-adds-crocs-to-impressive-list-of-nil-sponsors (October 30, 2022).

Gregory, Sean. "Chloe Kim Is Ready to Win Olympic Gold Again—on Her Own Terms." *Time*. 2022. https://time.com/6140099/chloe-kim-2022-olympics-snowboarder (May 4, 2022).

Griffith, Coleman Roberts. *Psychology of Coaching*. New York: Charles Scribner's Sons, 1926.

———. *Psychology of Athletics*. Champaign, IL: Bailey & Himes, 1927.

Gumbel, Bryant, host. *Real Sports with Bryant Gumbel*. Season 26, episode 10, "Episode 10." Aired November 24, 2020, in broadcast syndication. HBO, 2020, Vimeo.

Håkansson, Anders, Caroline Jönsson, and Göran Kenttä. "Psychological Distress and Problem Gambling in Elite Athletes during COVID-19 Restrictions—A Web Survey in Top Leagues of Three Sports during the Pandemic." *International Journal of Environmental Research and Public Health* 17, no. 18 (September 2020): 1–17.

Hensley-Clancy, Molly. "Reeling from Suicides, College Athletes Press NCAA: 'This Is a Crisis.'" *Washington Post*. 2022. https://www.washingtonpost.com/sports/2022/05/19/college-athletes-suicide-mental-health (October 30, 2022).

Hong, Eugene, and Ashwin L. Rao, eds. *Mental Health in the Athlete: Modern Perspectives and Novel Challenges for the Sports Medicine Provider*. Cham: Springer Nature, 2020.

"The Inside Story of a Toxic Culture at Maryland Football." *ESPN*. 2018. https://www.espn.com/college-football/story/_/id/24342005/maryland-terrapins-football-culture-toxic-coach-dj-durkin (March 5, 2022).

Jerkins, Morgan. "Naomi Osaka's Next Chapter." *Self*. 2022. https://www.self.com/story/naomi-osaka (May 9, 2022).

Jia, Lori, Michael V. Carter, Antonio Cusano, Xinning Li, John D. Kelly IV, Jessica D. Bartley, and Robert L. Parisien. "The Effect of the COVID-19 Pandemic on the Mental and Emotional Health of Athletes." *American Journal of Sports Medicine* 2022: 1–9.

Johnson, Greg. "NCAA Student-Athlete Well-Being Study." *NCAA*. 2022. https://www.ncaa.org/news/2022/5/24/media-center-mental-health-issues-remain-on-minds-of-student-athletes.aspx (May 26, 2022).

Kaplan, Emily. "NHL Reaches Settlement in Concussion Lawsuit." *ESPN*. 2018. https://www.espn.com/nhl/story/_/id/25256208/nhl-reaches-settlement-concussion-lawsuit (December 10, 2022).

Kearney, Audrey, Liz Hamel, and Mollyann Brodie. "Mental Health Impact of the COVID-19 Pandemic: An Update." *Kaiser Family Foundation*. 2021. https://www.kff.org/coronavirus-covid-19/poll-finding/mental-health-impact-of-the-covid-19-pandemic (July 27, 2022).

Kennedy, Merrit. "Simone Biles Withdraws from Individual All-Around Final at the Tokyo Olympics." *NPR*. 2021. https://www.npr.org/sections/tokyo-olympics-live-updates/2021/07/28/1021581409/simone-biles-withdraws-from-the-individual-all-around-final-at-tokyo-olympics (April 24, 2022).

Keown, Tim. "Discussing Mental Illness." *ESPN*. 2013. https://www.espn.com/nfl/story/_/id/9279525/meaningful-discussion-athletes-mental-illness (February 10, 2023).

Kilgore, Adam. "After Missing Olympics, Sha'Carri Richardson Remains in a Lane of Her Own." *Washington Post*. 2022. https://www.washingtonpost.com/sports/olympics/2022/06/21/shacarri-richardson-us-track-championships (December 24, 2022).

Kindelan, Katie. "Gymnastics Champion Simone Biles Reveals She Takes Anxiety Medication, Goes to Therapy after Speaking Out on Sexual Abuse." *Good Morning America*. 2018. https://www.goodmorningamerica.com/culture/story/gymnastics-champion-simone-biles-reveals-takes-anxiety-medicine-59746407 (April 24, 2022).

———. "Simone Biles Ties Mental Health Struggle at Tokyo Olympics to Nassar Sexual Abuse." *Good Morning America*. 2021. https://www.goodmorningamerica.com/wellness/story/simone-biles-ties-mental-health-struggle-tokyo-olympics-80038932 (December 29, 2022).

Kirkpatrick, Emily. "Naomi Osaka Tells Megyn Kelly to 'Do Better' after *Sports Illustrated* Criticism." *Vanity Fair*. 2021. https://www.vanityfair.com/style/2021/07/naomi-osaka-tells-megyn-kelly-do-better-critique-sports-illustrated-swimsuit-cover-after-withdraw-from-french-open (May 9, 2022).

Kliegman, Julie. "College Athletes Are Only Starting to Get Access to the Mental Health Care They Need." *The Ringer.* 2017. https://www.theringer.com/2017/10/26/16535274/ncaa-student-athletes-mental-health-care-initiatives (May 13, 2022).

———. "The State of Mental Health Care in the NBA." *The Ringer.* 2018. https://www.theringer.com/nba/2018/5/7/17320362/mental-health-nba (August 8, 2022).

———. "Sarah Fuller's Journey from Football Kicker to Mental Health Advocate." *Sports Illustrated.* 2022. https://www.si.com/college/2022/07/25/sarah-fuller-vanderbilt-football-daily-cover (October 30, 2022).

———. "Tough Breaks." *Sports Illustrated.* 2022. https://www.si.com/more-sports/2022/07/06/mental-toughness-the-strength-issue (November 6, 2022).

———. "Paddy Steinfort and the Craft of Mental Performance Coaching." *Sports Illustrated.* 2020. https://www.si.com/edge/2020/10/02/paddy-steinfort-mental-performance-coach-daily-cover (November 12, 2022).

———. "'Mentally, That's a Whole Nother Ball Game.'" *Sports Illustrated.* 2020. https://www.si.com/olympics/2020/04/29/mental-impact-of-the-pandemic-on-athletes (November 27, 2022).

———. "Michael Phelps on Mental Health and the USOPC: 'I Want People to Actually Do Something.'" *Sports Illustrated.* 2022. https://www.si.com/olympics/2015/11/09/michael-phelps-rehabilitation-rio-2016 (December 10, 2022).

———. "What Do Athletes Get from Ayahuasca, Mushrooms, and Ecstasy?" *Sports Illustrated.* 2022. https://www.si.com/more-sports/2022/08/12/psychedelics-sports-aaron-rodgers-daily-cover (December 25, 2022).

———. "Ben Simmons's Mental Health Is Not a Joke." *Sports Illustrated.* 2022. https://www.si.com/nba/2022/02/15/ben-simmons-mental-health-brooklyn-nets (January 6, 2023).

———. "'I Wasn't Really Doing It for Myself.'" *Sports Illustrated.* 2023. https://www.si.com/nba/2023/01/24/tyrell-terry-nba-stanford-retire-mental-health-daily-cover (February 4, 2023).

———. "Lolo Jones's Eternal Reinvention." *Sports Illustrated.* 2021. https://www.si.com/olympics/2021/07/07/where-are-they-now-lolo-jones (February 25, 2023).

Kornspan, Alan S., and Mary J. MacCracken. "Psychology Applied to Sport in the 1940s: The Work of Dorothy Hazeltine Yates." *The Sport Psychologist* 15 (2001): 342–45.

Kwiatkowski, Marisa, Mark Alesia, and Tim Evans. "A Blind Eye to Sex Abuse: How USA Gymnastics Failed to Report Cases." *Indianapolis Star.* 2016. https://www.indystar.com/story/news/investigations/2016/08/04/usa-gymnastics-sex-abuse-protected-coaches/85829732 (April 24, 2022).

Lawler, Jake. "A New Life." *Jake Lawler.* 2019. https://jakelawler.blog/2019/06/06/a-new-life (June 12, 2022).

Layden, Tim. "After Rehabilitation, the Best of Michael Phelps May Lie Ahead." *Sports Illustrated.* 2015. https://www.si.com/olympics/2015/11/09/michael-phelps-rehabilitation-rio-2016 (July 30, 2022).

Lee, Edward. "For UMBC Softball Star Courtney Coppersmith, Mental Health Is about Being 'More Than Just an Athlete.'" *Baltimore Sun.* 2022. https://www

.baltimoresun.com/sports/college/bs-sp-courtney-coppersmith-umbc-softball
-20220519-qzrfjzzedbfqpc636rrmpzg3iu-story.html (October 30, 2022).

Levenson, Eric. "Larry Nassar Apologizes, Gets 40 to 125 Years for Decades of Sexual
Abuse." *CNN.* 2018. https://www.cnn.com/2018/02/05/us/larry-nassar-sentence
-eaton/index.html (March 5, 2022).

Logue, Matt. "Shocking Details of Liz Cambage's Pre-Olympic Outburst Finally
Revealed." *Sunday Telegraph.* 2022. https://www.news.com.au/sport/basketball/liz
-cambage-called-nigerian-players-monkeys-slapped-rival-in-the-face/news-story
/013353c7eabbc113b56cbc35ddeaa628 (October 15, 2022).

Lundgren, Tobias, Gustaf Reinebo, Per Olov-Löf, Markus Näslund, Per Svartvadet, and
Thomas Parling. "The Values, Acceptance, and Mindfulness Scale for Ice Hockey
Players." *Frontiers in Psychology* 9, no. 1794 (October 2018), https://doi.org/10.3389
/fpsyg.2018.01794.

MacMullan, Jackie. "When Making the NBA Isn't a Cure-All: Mental Health and Black
Athletes." *ESPN.* 2018. https://www.espn.com/nba/story/_/id/24393541/jackie
-macmullan-complex-issue-mental-health-nba-african-american-community
(February 10, 2023).

"Major Depression." *National Institute of Mental Health.* 2022. https://www.nimh.nih.gov
/health/statistics/major-depression (March 5, 2022).

Mandel, Stewart. "College Football Recruits Signing 6- and 7-Figure NIL Deals as
Market Grows." *The Athletic.* 2022. https://theathletic.com/3500422/2022/04
/19/college-football-recruits-signing-6-and-7-figure-nil-deals-as-market-grows
(October 30, 2022).

Marshall, Ashley. "Naomi Osaka Defeats Serena Williams in Dramatic Final." *U.S. Open.*
2018. https://www.usopen.org/en_US/news/articles/2018-09-08/naomi_osaka_
derails_serena_williams_in_dramatic_final.html (April 12, 2022).

Marwell, Emet. "Former Hockey Player Emet Marwell: The Impossible Choice of Passion or Truth." *Athlete Ally.* 2019. http://www.athleteally.org/emet-marwell-the
-impossible-choice (July 28, 2022).

May, Jerry R., and Michael J. Asken, eds. *Sport Psychology: The Psychological Health of the
Athlete.* New York: PMA Publishing Corporation, 1987.

McCallie, Joanne P. *Secret Warrior: A Coach and Fighter, On and Off the Court.* Virginia
Beach, VA: Koehler Books, 2021.

McCarvel, Nick. "Gracie 3.0: Olympian Gold Eyes 'Big Goals' in Continued Comeback."
Olympics. 2022. https://olympics.com/en/news/gracie-gold-2014-olympian-big
-goals-comeback-figure-skating (February 26, 2023).

"McKayla Maroney Is Not Impressed." *Know Your Meme.* 2012. https://knowyourmeme
.com/memes/mckayla-is-not-impressed (March 5, 2022).

"McKayla Maroney Selling 'Not Impressed' NFT." *TMZ.* 2021. https://www.tmz.com
/2021/08/10/mckayla-maroney-selling-not-impressed-nft-olympics-viral-image
-meme (March 5, 2022).

Mechikoff, Robert, with Virginia Evans. *Sport Psychology for Women.* New York: Harper-
Collins, 1987.

"Mental Health Best Practices." *NCAA Sport Science Institute.* 2016. http://s3.amazonaws
.com/ncaa.org/documents/2021/1/18/HS_Mental_Health_Best_Practices
_20160317.pdf (July 25, 2022).

Merryweather, Alice, as told to Megan Soisson. "In Her Own Words: Alice Merryweather
Details Eating Disorder Treatment." *NBC Sports.* 2021. https://onherturf.nbcsports
.com/2021/03/16/alpine-skier-alice-merryweather-eating-disorder-treatment-in
-her-own-words (February 10, 2023).

Metzl, Jonathan M., and Kenneth T. MacLeish. "Mental Illness, Mass Shootings, and
the Politics of American Firearms." *American Journal of Public Health* 105, no. 2
(February 2015): 240–49.

Miller Aron, Cindy, Sydney Harvey, Brian Hainline, Mary E. Hitchcock, and Claudia
Reardon. "Post-Traumatic Stress Disorder (PTSD) and Other Trauma-Related
Mental Health Disorders in Elite Athletes: A Narrative Review." *British Journal of
Sports Medicine* 53, no. 12 (June 2019): 779–84.

Mizoguchi, Karen. "Timeline of Simone Biles' Tokyo Olympics: From Skipping Opening
Ceremony to Exiting Her Event Finals." *People.* 2021. https://people.com/sports/
tokyo-olympics-simone-biles-timeline-withdrawals-event-finals/#6c64fab2-0a4e
-47bf-aa57-d61fc8d06446 (May 1, 2022).

Murphy, Geraldine, Albert J. Pepitas, and Britton W. Brewer. "Identity Foreclosure,
Athletic Identity, and Career Maturity in Intercollegiate Athletes." *The Sport Psychologist* 10, no. 3 (1996): 239–46.

NCAA, Twitter post, March 15, 2021, 9 p.m. https://twitter.com/ncaa/status
/1371627276899520514?lang=en (May 22, 2022).

"NCAA National Study on Substance Use Habits of College Student-Athletes."
NCAA. 2018. https://ncaaorg.s3.amazonaws.com/research/substance/2017RES
_SubstanceUseExecutiveSummary.pdf (December 25, 2022).

"NCAA Student-Athlete Well-being Study." *NCAA.* 2022. https://www.ncaa.org/news
/2022/5/24/media-center-mental-health-issues-remain-on-minds-of-student
-athletes.aspx (May 26, 2022).

Niesen, Joan. "In a Divided US, It's No Surprise Some See Simone Biles as a Villain."
The Guardian. 2021. https://www.theguardian.com/sport/2021/jul/28/simone-biles
-withdrawal-olympics-gymnastics-tokyo-media-reaction (May 1, 2022).

Olivieri, Anthony. "Metta World Peace Opens Up about His Mental Health Journey
and the Importance of Therapy." 2021. https://www.espn.com/nba/story/_/id
/31472342/metta-world-peace-opens-mental-health-journey-importance-therapy
(February 10, 2023).

Olney, Buster. "Troubled Harnisch Put on Disabled List." *New York Times.* 1997. https:
//www.nytimes.com/1997/04/08/sports/troubled-harnisch-put-on-disabled-list
.html (December 9, 2022).

Osaka, Naomi. "Naomi Osaka: 'It's O.K. to Not Be O.K.'" *Time.* 2021. https://time.com
/6077128/naomi-osaka-essay-tokyo-olympics (May 5, 2022).

Panchal, Nirmita, Rabah Kamal, Cynthia Cox, and Rachel Garfield. "The Implications of COVID-19 for Mental Health and Substance Use." *Kaiser Family*

Foundation. 2021. https://www.kff.org/report-section/the-implications-of-covid-19-for-mental-health-and-substance-use-issue-brief (July 27, 2022).

Park, Alice. "How Olympians Are Fighting to Put Athletes' Mental Health First." *Time.* 2021. https://time.com/6082203/tokyo-olympics-mental-health (February 10, 2023).

Patterson, Orlando. *Slavery and Social Death.* Cambridge, MA: Harvard University Press, 1982.

Penn, Nate. "How to Build the Perfect Batter." *GQ.* September 2006, 292–305.

Perna, F., J. Roh, R. Newcomer, and E. F. Etzel. "Clinical Depression among Injured Athletes: An Empirical Assessment." *Association for the Advancement of Applied Sport Psychology Annual Convention.* 1998.

Pianovich, Stephen. "Roger Federer Pulls Out of 2021 French Open: 'It's Important That I Listen to My Body.'" *CBS Sports.* 2021. https://www.cbssports.com/tennis/news/roger-federer-pulls-out-of-2021-french-open-its-important-that-i-listen-to-my-body (May 9, 2022).

Piersall, Jimmy. *Fear Strikes Out.* Lincoln, NE: Bison Books, 1999.

Pilkington, Vita, Simon M. Rice, Courtney C. Walton, Kate Gwyther, Lisa Olive, Matt Butterworth, Matti Clements, Gemma Cross, and Rosemary Purcell. "Prevalence and Correlates of Mental Health Symptoms and Well-Being among Elite Sport Coaches and High-Performance Support Staff." *Sports Medicine Open* 8, no. 1 (July 2022): 89.

Powell, Jackie. "The WNBA Is Finally Catching Up on Mental Health." *Sports Illustrated.* 2021. https://www.si.com/wnba/2021/08/19/mental-health-illness-wnbpa-speaking-out (October 15, 2022).

"Psychology of Athletics Will Be Tried at Illinois." *New York Times.* April 2, 1922, 30.

Puhl, Rebeca M., Janet D. Latner, Kelly M. King, and Joerg Luedicke. "Weight Bias among Professionals Treating Eating Disorders: Attitudes about Treatment and Perceived Patient Outcomes." *International Journal of Eating Disorders* 47, no. 1 (January 2014): 65–75.

Purna Kambhampaty, Anna. "The Surprising—and Sometimes Troubling—History of Tennis Clothes." 2019. https://time.com/5667447/tennis-clothes-history (March 5, 2022).

Purtell, Laura M., and Anna Katherine Clemmons. "Athlete-Mom Confidential: How the Pros Manage Motherhood." *ESPN.* 2018. https://www.espn.com/espnw/story/_/id/24528874/athlete-mom-confidential-how-pros-manage-motherhood (October 11, 2022).

Ramsay, George, and Don Riddell, "Bianca Andreescu: How a Fake Check Inspired the U.S. Open Champion," *CNN.* 2019. https://www.cnn.com/2019/09/08/tennis/bianca-andreescu-us-open-serena-williams-tennis-spt-intl (November 12, 2022).

Rao, Ashwin L., Irfan M. Asif, Jonathan A. Drezner, Brett G. Toresdahl, and Kimberly G. Harmon. "Suicide in National Collegiate Athletic Association (NCAA) Athletes: A 9-Year Analysis of the NCAA Resolutions Database." *Sports Health* 7, no. 5 (September 2015): 452–57.

Rapkin, Brett, director. *The Weight of Gold*. HBO, 2020. 1 hour. https://www.hbo.com/movies/the-weight-of-gold.

Reardon, Claudia L., Abhinav Bindra, Cheri Blauwet, Richard Budgett, Niccolo Campriani, Alan Currie, Vincent Gouttebarge, David McDuff, Margo Mountjoy, Rosemary Purcell, Margot Putukian, Simon Rice, and Brian Hainline. "Mental Health Management of Elite Athletes during COVID-19: A Narrative Review and Recommendations." *British Journal of Sports Medicine* no. 55 (September 2020): 608–15.

Rhoden, William C. "With No One Looking, a Hurt Stays Hidden." *New York Times*. 2012. https://www.nytimes.com/2012/10/30/sports/with-no-one-looking-mental-illness-in-athletes-can-stay-hidden.html (February 10, 2023).

Ricci, Taylor, and Nathan Braaten, "Pac-12 Grant Awardee Final Report." *Dam Worth It*. 2021.

Richmond, Sam. "1st College Football Game Ever Was New Jersey vs. Rutgers in 1869." *NCAA*. 2019. https://www.ncaa.com/news/football/article/2017-11-06/college-football-history-heres-when-1st-game-was-played (March 5, 2022).

Robson, Dan. "'We're All Hurting, We Need Answers': Why Former Pro Athletes Are Leading the 'Psychedelic Revolution.'" *The Athletic*. 2021. https://theathletic.com/2625498/2021/06/04/were-all-hurting-we-need-answers-why-former-pro-athletes-are-leading-the-psychedelic-revolution (February 7, 2023).

Roenigk, Alyssa. "Why Simone Biles Withdrew from the Olympic Women's Gymnastics Team Final—'You Have to Be 100%.'" *ESPN*. 2021. https://www.espn.com/olympics/story/_/id/31897727/why-simone-biles-withdrew-team-final-be-100-percent (April 24, 2022).

———. "Lotus Pose on Two." *ESPN*. 2013. https://www.espn.com/nfl/story/_/id/9581925/seattle-seahawks-use-unusual-techniques-practice-espn-magazine (February 10, 2023).

"Roosevelt Praises Boxing." *New York Times*. May 9, 1913, 3.

Russo, Ralph D. "ACC, Big Ten, Pac 12 Launch Mental Health Initiative." *Associated Press*. 2021. https://apnews.com/article/sports-health-mens-college-basketball-college-basketball-mental-health-beb493e5f0dba62e052634720b1c9880 (October 30, 2022).

Sabathia, CC, and Chris Smith. *Till the End*. New York: Roc Lit 101, 2021.

Salahi, Lara. "Catherine Zeta-Jones Sheds Light on Bipolar II Disorder." *ABC*. 2011. https://abcnews.go.com/Health/BipolarDisorder/catherine-zeta-jones-sheds-light-bipolar-disorder/story?id=13373202 (July 17, 2022).

Sanchez, Robert. "Dirty Pool at the Paralympics: Will Cheating Ruin the Games?" *Sports Illustrated*. 2020. https://www.si.com/olympics/2020/03/03/paralympiccheating (November 12, 2022).

Scurry, Briana, and Wayne Coffey. *My Greatest Save: The Brave, Barrier-Breaking Journey of a World-Champion Goalkeeper*. New York: Abrams Press, 2022.

Seidel, Molly, as told to Charlotte Gibson. "How Olympic Runner Molly Seidel Found a Way to Run Again." *ESPN*. 2021. https://www.espn.com/olympics/story/_/page/

Going-September252020/how-olympic-marathoner-molly-seidel-found-way-run -again (April 10, 2022).

Seles, Monica. *Getting a Grip: On My Body, My Mind, My Self.* New York: Avery, 2010.

Smith, Doug. "Williams' Father Says Booing Was Racially Motivated." *USA Today.* 2001. http://usatoday30.usatoday.com/sports/tennis/stories/2001-03-26-williams .htm (May 5, 2022).

Sneed, Brandon. *Head in the Game: The Mental Engineering of the World's Greatest Athletes.* New York: HarperCollins, 2017.

Sudano, Laura E., Greg Collins, and Christopher M. Miles, "Reducing Barriers to Mental Health Care for Student-Athletes: An Integrated Care Model," *Families, Systems, and Health* 35, no. 1 (2017): 77–84.

Sudano, Laura E., and Christopher M. Miles, "Mental Health Services in NCAA Division I Athletics: A Survey of Head ATCs," *Sports Health* 9, no. 3 (May–June 2017): 262–67.

Svoboda, Elizabeth. "An Athletic Coach for the Mind?" *New York Times.* 2021. https:// www.nytimes.com/2021/08/05/well/move/mental-skills-coaching-olympics.html (February 10, 2023).

Svrluga, Barry. "An Olympic Skier's Battle with Anorexia: 'I Didn't Really Realize I Had a Problem.'" *Washington Post.* 2021. https://www.washingtonpost.com/sports/2021 /03/10/alice-merryweather-anorexia-olympics-skiing (February 7, 2023).

"Tackling Mental Health in Olympic Sport." *International Olympic Committee.* 2019. https: //olympics.com/ioc/news/tackling-mental-health-in-olympic-sport (February 27, 2022).

Tarkan, Laurie. "Athletes' Injuries Go beyond the Physical." *New York Times.* 2000. https: //www.nytimes.com/2000/09/26/health/athletes-injuries-go-beyond-the-physical .html (February 10, 2023).

Theberge, Nancy, and Peter Donnelly, eds. *Sport and the Sociological Imagination.* Fort Worth: Texas Christian University Press, 1984.

Tracy, David F. *The Psychologist at Bat.* New York: Sterling Publishing, 1951.

Triplett, Norman. "The Dynamogenic Factors in Pacemaking and Competition." *American Journal of Psychology* 9, no. 4 (July 1898): 507–33.

Tyrrell, Patrick, Seneca Harberger, Caroline Schoo, and Wadquar Siddiqui. "Kubler-Ross Stages of Dying and Subsequent Models of Grief." *National Library of Medicine.* 2022. https://www.ncbi.nlm.nih.gov/books/NBK507885 (July 27, 2022).

Van Raalte, Judy L., and Britton W. Brewer, eds. *Exploring Sport and Exercise Psychology.* Washington, DC: American Psychological Association, 1996.

Veeck, Bill, and Ed Linn. *Veeck—As in Wreck: The Autobiography of Bill Veeck.* Chicago: University of Chicago Press, 1962.

Walton, Courtney C., and Liknaitzky, Paul. "Advancing Elite Athlete Mental Health Treatment with Psychedelic-Assisted Psychotherapy." *Journal of Applied Sport Psychology* 34, no. 3 (2022): 605–23.

Welch, Bob, and George Vecsey. *Five O'Clock Comes Early: A Young Man's Battle with Alcoholism.* New York: William Morrow, 1981.

Williams, Jean M., ed. *Applied Sport Psychology: Personal Growth to Peak Performance*. 8th ed. New York: McGraw Hill, 2020.

Wolanin, Andrew, Eugene Hong, Donald Marks, Kelly Panchoo, and Michael Gross. "Prevalence of Clinically Elevated Depressive Symptoms in College Athletes and Differences by Gender and Sport." *British Journal of Sports Medicine* 50, no. 3 (January 2016): 167–71.

INDEX

Abad-Santos, Alex, 101
Abramowicz, Daria, 45–46
abuse: anxiety and depression
   from, 12; emotional abuse,
   14–15; sexual assault and, 11,
   12, 103–4, 127, 139
adaptive equipment, 50
American Journal of Psychology, 22
*American Journal of Sports
   Medicine*, 102
American Psychological
   Association Division 47, 38
Andreescu, Bianca, 48–49, 109–11
Angel City FC, 94
Angle, Paul M., 29, 30
anorexia nervosa, 160. *See also*
   eating disorders
Anthony, Carmelo, 8–10
antidepressants, 151
anxiety: abuse leading to, 12;
   awareness movement, 88;
   Biles's disclosures about,
   103–4; medication for, 69; at
   retirement, 184–85; substance
   use and, 145; support for
   players with, 83, 87; symptoms

of anxiety, 67–69. *See also*
   depression
Apstein, Stephanie, 105
"arm-chair psychologists," 23
Association for Applied Sport
   Psychology, 38
Astor, Maggie, 170
Athlete Ally advocacy group, 182
Athlete EDGE Program, 174, 175
athlete identity foreclosure,
   8–10, 124
athletes of color, xxii, 9, 36–37,
   101–2
Athletics Research Laboratory,
   26–27
Atlanta Braves, 40–41
Atlanta Dream, 63
Axelrod, David, 74–75

Bader, LaTisha, 56, 144–45
Bailar, Schuyler, 167, 174, 175
Balcer, Bethany, 93–94
Ball Four (Bouton), 189
Bannon, Steve, 73
Bartley, Jessica, 112–14, 174
Barty, Ash, 99
Bauman, Jim, 7

Beard, Amanda, 162–63, 164, 171, 174
beginnings of sport psychology: conferences, 23–24; early journals/studies, 21–24, 38; gender bias in, 34–37; Griffith's work, 25–30; role of race in, 36–37; seriousness of the field, xx, 37–38; study of Babe Ruth, 24–25; Tracy's work, 30–34
Beijing Games, 112
Bell, Mariah, 185
Benjamin, Ludy T., 37–38
Bennett, Gary, 121–23, 177–78
Bennett, Kate, 161–62, 167, 172, 174, 176
Bernett, Lauren, 131
Betchart, Graham, 186
Bieber, Justin, 107
Biles, Simone: comeback, 105–6; disclosures of, 10, 103–4; during pandemic, 186–87; performance issues, xv, 55–56; reactions to, 101–2, 106–7; withdrawing from events, 104–5
binge drinking, 142, 143
binge eating, 160
bipolar disorder, xvii–xviii, 61–62, 64, 84, 182
Black athletes. See athletes of color
Blindsided podcast, 90
BMI (body mass index), 162, 168
body image. See eating disorders

body mass index (BMI), 162, 168
Bouton, Jim, 189
Braaten, Nathan, 12, 133–34
Bradley, Bill, 189
brain conditions, 4, 140–41, 156
Buffalo Beauts, 179
bulimia nervosa, 160. See also eating disorders
Bull, Andy, 75

Cain, Mary, 169–70
Cambage, Liz, 88–89
Canadian teams, 107–9, 113–14, 139
cannabis consumption, 143–45
Carcillo, Daniel, 139–41, 149–50, 152–54
Carpenter, Carrie, 50–52
Carr, Chris, xx, 9, 45, 56, 92
Carter, Jennifer, 162, 165, 168–69
Carter, Leeja, 34
Carter-Francique, Akilah, xxii, 9–10, 102
CBA (collective bargaining agreement), 93–94
Centre College, 178
Chen, Anelise, 189–90
Chicago Bulls, 83
Chicago Cubs, 28–30
Chicago White Sox, 191–92
chronic traumatic encephalopathy (CTE), 4, 140–41, 156
Cincinnati Reds, 67
Clarendon, Layshia, xxii–xxiii, 15, 84, 187–88

classification of Paralympians, 50
Cleveland Cavaliers, 81, 187
coaches: eating disorders
    influenced by, 168–70;
    perfectionism and, 14–15;
    role in mental health, 14–16;
    sexual abuse by, 11, 12,
    103–4, 107. See also mental
    performance coaches
Coffey, Wayne, 143, 188
cognitive defusion, 52
collective bargaining agreement
    (CBA), 93–94
collegiate mental
    health: awareness campaigns,
    127–29; counseling methods,
    16; dedicated practitioners,
    121–23; at Division I level,
    127–28; football as war
    metaphor, 5–6; grassroots
    dialogue, 132–34; pressures
    in sports, 123–27; resources
    for, 115, 118–21; services for
    veterans of athletics, 135;
    stigma of mental illness,
    127–29; substance use, 143. See
    also National Association of
    Intercollegiate Athletics
    (NAIA); National Collegiate
    Athletic Association (NCAA)
Collins, Greg, 123
Conboy, Sean Patrick, 86–88
concussions, 140–41
confidentiality, 55
Connecticut Sun, 187–88

Connole, Ian, 118, 129, 132
Conviser, Jenny, 163–64
Coppersmith, Courtney, 131
Coubertin, Pierre de, 23
Court, Rick, 6–7
COVID-19 pandemic, xix–xx,
    95–96, 102–3, 109–10, 111–12,
    130, 185–87
CTE (chronic traumatic
    encephalopathy), 4, 140–
    41, 156
cyclists, studies of, 22–23

Dallas Mavericks, 40
Dallas Wings, 85
Dames, Rory, 94
Dam Worth It campaign, 12–13,
    84, 133–34
Danz, Hailey, 49–50
Dartmouth sports, 191
Delayo, Mike, 18–19, 86, 91
Denver Broncos, 180
depression: abuse leading to,
    12; collegiate athletes and,
    7–8; DeRozan's disclosure,
    79–80; Harnisch's disclosure,
    65–66; injured athletes and,
    179; as ongoing struggle, 87;
    Osaka's disclosure, 100–101;
    postpartum, 85. See also anxiety;
    Phelps, Michael; suicide
DeRozan, DeMar, 10, 70, 79–80,
    82–86, 89, 95–96

Diagnostic and Statistical Manual of Mental Disorders (DSM-5), xxi, 160
Diggins-Smith, Skylar, 85
digital media, 86–89, 91–92. *See also* Instagram stories; *The Players' Tribune*
disabled list/injured list, 65–66
Dorfman, Harvey, 41–42
Dorpfeld, Lee, 141–43, 144, 149
Durkin, DJ, 6–7

eating disorders: about, 159–62; coaches' role in, 168–70; gender issues, 165–66; media and social media influencing, 170–72; queer athletes and, 166–67; risk factors, 164–65; treatments, 172–76; weight bias and, 162–64
ecstasy (MDMA), 153, 155
emotional abuse, 14–15
Evans, Rashad, 151–52, 153
evolution of sports, 37–38

Fader, Mirin, 87
Fagan, Kate, xx, 10, 15–16, 123, 125, 130, 135–36, 178
FDA (Food and Drug Administration), 153
Federer, Roger, 101
Feldpausch, Nora, 121
Felix, Camonghne, 104
Feltz, Deborah L., 36

Feminist Applied Sport Psychology (Carter), 34
fencers, studies of, 23
field hockey, 182–83
Field Trip, 152
fight-or-flight response, 8
figure skating, 184–85
Fishbein, Jeffrey, 186, 191–92
Five O'Clock Comes Early (Welch), 148–49
Floyd, George, 72
focus, 39
Food and Drug Administration (FDA), 153
football deaths, 6–7
football metaphor for mental health dialogue, 73
Freakley, Ben, 52–54
French Open, 98–101
Frontiers in Psychology study, 47
Fuller, Sarah, 125
Fullerton, Hugh S., 24–25

Gajewski, Kenny, 131
games, 51
Garden, Greg, 178
Gaudiani, Jennifer "Dr. G," 162, 163, 166–67, 176
gender issues: female athletes and depression, 7; gender bias, 34–37; LGBTQ+ concerns, xxi–xxii, 166–67, 182–83; media coverage of women, 89–90; men and eating disorders, 165–66

Generation K, 67–70
Gervais, Michael, 8, 43–44, 191
Getting a Grip (Seles), 171–72
Gill, Diane L., 34–35, 36
Gobert, Rudy, 185
Gold, Gracie, 106, 162
Golenbock, Peter, 28–29
Gottlieb, Doug, 106
Goucher, Kara, 169–70
Green, Christopher D., 22, 27, 29–30
Green Bay Packers, 92
grief, xviii, 181
Griffith, Coleman Roberts, 25–30
Grimm, Charlie, 28, 29
Gunter, Kensa, 178, 186
gymnastics, 104–5, 110. *See also specific athletes*

Hacker, Colleen, 42
Hainline, Brian, 4, 11, 14, 119–20, 127–28, 130, 132
Hall, Ruth, 36–37
Hamm, Mia, 13
Harnisch, Pete, 65–67, 76–77
Harris, Dorothy V., 35–36
Hartnett, Gabby, 29
Hayes, Steven C., 44–45, 46–47, 56–57
health insurance, 113
Henrich, Christy, 170
Hilinski, Tyler (and family), 3–4, 15, 121, 123, 126, 129–30
Hilinski's Hope Foundation, 4, 129

Hill, Jayden, 131
Hill, Jemele, 106
Hirsch, Corey, 90–91
hockey players, 47
Holcomb, Steven, 75–76
Holdsclaw, Chamique, 61–65
Holleran, Madison, 10, 125, 130, 136
Holmes, Joseph, 24–25
Houston Rockets, 70–71
Huff, George, 26

identity foreclosure, 8–10
Indianapolis Colts, 85–86
individual model of sport psychology, 46–47
injuries, 182–83. *See also* time-off from games
Instagram stories, 100, 105, 107, 170–71
internal monologues, 39, 51
International Journal of Eating Disorders, 163
International Journal of Sport Psychology, 38
In the Water They Can't See You Cry (Beard), 174

Jackson, Kalen, 85
Jackson, Terri, 89
James, LeBron, xxiii, 21, 84, 199
James Madison University softball, 131
The Jed Foundation, 126, 127
Jenkins, Sally, 62

Jerkins, Morgan, 101
Johanson, Albert, 24–25
Johnson, Matthew W., 151, 157
Jones, Lolo, 17–18
Journal of Applied Sport Psychology, 181
Journal of Sport Psychology, 38

Kaiser Family Foundation (KFF), 185
Kalkstein, Don, 40, 45
Katz, Jonathan F., 40–41, 45
Kennedy Forum conference, 75
Kerr, Steve, 84
Kessler, Gabby, 94
ketamine, 151, 152–53, 155
KFF (Kaiser Family Foundation), 185
Kicking the Stigma campaign, 85–86
Kim, Chloe, 111–12
King, Billie Jean, 99, 100–101, 111
Kirk, Charlie, 106
Kornspan, Alan, 30, 35, 36
Kübler-Ross, Elisabeth, 181

Labbé, Stephanie, 107–9
Las Vegas Aces, 64–65
Lawler, Jake, 120, 126, 132–33
Leach, Mike, 129
Lego builds, 51
Lehner, Robin, 84
Leonard, Shaquille, 86
Lerch, Stephen, 189
Levy, Ronan, 152

LGBTQ+ athletes, xxi–xxii, 166–67, 182–83
Life on the Run (Bradley), 189
Light (documentary), 165
Liknaitzky, Paul, 150
Lipsyte, Robert, 67
Littwin, Mike, 41
Llewellyn, Jack, 41
Los Angeles Sparks, 63
Love, Kevin: advice from, 187; disclosures of, 70, 72–73, 81–83, 88, 89; reactions to, 83–86; sparking movement, 95–96
Lynch, Marshawn, 98–99

MAC (Mid-American Conference), 128–29
MacPhee, John, 126, 127
Mad Pride movement, xx–xxi
"mad traveler," 22
magic mushrooms (psilocybin), 141, 149–51, 152, 153–54, 155
Major League Baseball (MLB), 155. *See also specific teams and players*
Maller, Ben, 106
Mantra Health, 121
Marjama, Mike, 165–66, 174
Marks, Gabe, 117–18, 120, 129–30, 135
Marmol, Oliver, 15
Maroney, McKayla, 10–12
Martin, Robert, 131
Marwell, Emet, 143, 182–83

Mayo Clinic, 181
McConville, Rebecca, 160, 168, 171, 175
McDuff, David R., 145, 146, 148
McKinley, Kenny, 180–81
McNair, Jordan, 6
MDMA (ecstasy), 153, 155
media: digital media, 86–89, 91–92; Instagram stories, 100, 105, 107, 170–71; press conferences, 97–99, 114; reactions to athletes' disclosures, 83–86, 100–102, 106–7; social media attention, 12, 124–25
meditation. *See* mindfulness and meditation
mental health: accommodations for, 70–72; benefits of toughness, 5; illness as taboo, 61; mental illness vs., xx–xxi; mental performance and, 55–57; pressing questions about, xxii–xxiii; sharing struggles, 16–19; vulnerability and, xxiv. *See also* anxiety; beginnings of sport psychology; bipolar disorders; depression; pioneers in mental health and sports
mental performance coaches: about, xxiii–xxiv; clinicians compared to, 44–46; early days of using, 39–42; explosion of field, 42–44; teammates working together

with, 53–54; working one-on-one with, 54–55
Merryweather, Alice, 159–60, 168, 173–74
Meyer, Katie, 130–31
Mid-American Conference (MAC), 128–29
Miles, Christopher M., 123
Milwaukee Bucks, 87
Mind, Body and Sport guide (NCAA), 179–80
mindfulness and meditation: about, xxiii–xxiv; Andreescu's visualization, 48–49; benefits, 47, 49; exercises, 53; training in, 40
MIT Sloan Sports Analytics Conference, 93
MLB (Major League Baseball), 155. *See also specific teams and players*
Montador, Steve, 140, 141
Morgan, Piers, 99
Morse, Mackenzie, 13–14, 161, 177, 191
Mount Holyoke field hockey, 182–83
Murphy, Chris, 50
My Greatest Save (Scurry and Coffey), 143, 188

Nadal, Rafael, 99
NAIA (National Association of Intercollegiate Athletics), 121

name, image, and likeness (NIL), 124, 125–26
Nassar, Larry, 11, 12, 103–4, 107
Nassib, Carl, xxi–xxii
National Association of Intercollegiate Athletics (NAIA), 121
National Basketball Association (NBA), 92–93, 141–42, 145, 155. *See also specific teams and players*
National Collegiate Athletic Association (NCAA): interpersonal relationships among athletes, 136; mental health best practices, 119; *Mind, Body and Sport* guide, 179–80; retirement of student athletes, 126–27; room for growth in, 134–35; substance use, 143; suicides, 129–32; transfer regulations, 126. *See also* Hainline, Brian; *specific teams and players*
National Football League (NFL), 92, 145. *See also specific teams and players*
National Hockey League (NHL), 139–41, 146. *See also specific teams and players*
National Women's Hockey League (NWHL), 179
National Women's Soccer League (NWSL), 14, 93–95. *See also specific teams and players*

NBA (National Basketball Association), 92–93, 141–42, 145, 155. *See also specific teams and players*
NCAA. *See* National Collegiate Athletic Association (NCAA)
Neumann, Kelsey, 16–17, 19, 179
New York Islanders, 84
New York Liberty draft, 102
New York Rangers, 40
NFL (National Football League), 92, 145. *See also specific teams and players*
NHL (National Hockey League), 139–41, 146. *See also specific teams and players*
Nicholson, Josie, 16, 122, 123–24, 129, 130
Nickols, Riley, 161, 166, 169–70, 174
NIL (name, image, and likeness), 124, 125–26
NOCAP Sports, 125
"not impressed" expression, 11–12
Novitzky, Jeff, 154
NWHL (National Women's Hockey League), 179
NWSL (National Women's Soccer League), 14, 93–95. *See also specific teams and players*

Oakland Athletics, 41
obsessive–compulsive disorder (OCD), 90–91
Ocasio-Cortez, Alexandria, 107

OCD (obsessive–compulsive disorder), 90–91

Oglesby, Carole, 36

Ogwumike, Nneka, 93

Olympics: in Athens, 75; in Beijing, 112; Coubertin on, 23; drug testing, 144; eating disorders and, 162–63; post-Games comedown, 49; in PyeongChang, 166; severe lows after, xv–xvii; in Tokyo, xix–xx, 89, 105, 107, 111–12, 186–87; USOPC, 38, 112–14, 178, 184–85; *The Weight of Gold* documentary, 17–18, 75–76, 113. *See also specific Olympic athletes*

Oregon State University, 133–34

orthorexia, 161. *See also* eating disorders

Osaka, Naomi, xv, 10, 97–102, 104, 114–15

Oubre, Kelly, Jr., 83

pandemic. *See* COVID-19 pandemic

panic attacks, 81, 88, 94

Paralympians, 49–50

Patterson, Orlando, 188

Penn, Nate, 25

perfectionism, 10–15, 164

Phelps, Michael: alcohol use, 146–47; on Biles, 106–7; disclosers of, xv, 74–76; on USOPC, 114; *The Weight of Gold* (documentary), 17, 75–76, 113

Philip K. Wrigley (Angle), 29, 30

Pilon, Mary, 70

pioneers in mental health and sports: Chamique Holdsclaw, 61–65; Bill Pulsipher, 61, 67–70; Pete Harnisch, 61, 65–67; Royce White, 61. *See also* beginnings of sport psychology

The Players' Tribune, 72–73, 81, 86–89, 90

Plummer, Jake, 155–56

Poland's lack of regulation, 46

Poneman, Daniel, 150–54

Postgraduate Medical Journal, 163

post-traumatic stress disorder (PTSD), 9–10, 84, 127

Powell, Jackie, 89

practice, 48

Prescott, Dak, 10

present moment awareness, 53

Press, Christen, 94

press conferences, 97–99, 114

privilege, xxii

professional sports leagues, 92–95. *See also specific leagues*

psilocybin (magic mushrooms), 141, 149–51, 152, 153–54, 155

psychedelics: athletes' use of, 154–57; ayahuasca, 154–55; FDA approval of, 153–54; help and harm from, 156–57; ketamine, 151, 152–54, 155;

MDMA, 153, 155; psilocybin, 141, 149–51, 152, 153–54, 155; relief gained from, 152
psychiatric medicine, 66, 150–52
"Psychological Observations Concerned with a Cycling Record" (Tissié), 23
Psychology Gets in the Game (Green and Benjamin), 21–22, 37–38
Psychology of Adjustment course, 35
Psychology of Coaching (Griffith), 26
PTSD (post-traumatic stress disorder), 9–10, 84, 127
Pulsipher, Bill, 67–70
PyeongChang Olympics, 166

queer athletes, xxi–xxii, 166–67, 182–83

racial issues, xxii, 9, 36–37, 101–2
Rago, Maria, 170
reactions to disclosures, 83–86, 100–102, 106–7. See also specific players
Real Sports, 154
The Reappearing Act (Fagan), 10
Reardon, Claudia, 119, 142
rehabilitation/treatment centers, 140, 147–49, 173–76, 182–83
Reitz, Aaron, 106
relationship building, 51–52
retirement of athletes, 16–17, 141, 184–85, 188–91

Reviving Baseball in Inner Cities organization, 131–32
Ricci, Taylor, 12–13, 84, 133–34
Richards, DiDi, 102, 121
Richardson, Sha'Carri, 144
The Ringer, 70, 73, 87, 88, 121, 122, 141
Rio Olympics, xix, 49, 103, 108
Rippon, Adam, 107, 166, 184–85
Rodgers, Aaron, 92, 154–55
Roosevelt, Teddy, 23
Rosenberg, Edwin, 188, 191
Rubenking, Erin, 142, 145
Ruth, George Herman, Jr. (Babe), 24–25

Sabathia, CC, 147–49
Salazar, Alberto, 169–70
Samuelson, Katie Lou, 102
San Antonio Silver Stars, 64–65
Sanders, Larry, 87
Saunders, Raven "the Hulk," xv–xvii
Schuck, Raymond I., 65–66, 76–77
Scripture, Edward Wheeler, 22, 23
Scurry, Briana, 42, 143, 188
Seattle Mariners, 165–66
Seattle Seahawks, 44, 98–99
Seattle Storm, 182
Seidel, Molly, 175
Seles, Monica, 171–72
self-medication, 142–43
The Separator (handbook), 52–53

sexual assault and abuse, 11, 12, 103–4, 127, 139
Sheahan, Riley, 146
Shulze, Sarah, 131
The Sideline Perspective (blog), 177
Silver, Adam, 93
Simmerling, Georgia, 108–9
Singer, Robert, 37
Skidmore basketball, 118
Smith, Chris, 147
Smith, Doug, 80
Smoltz, John, 40–41
snowboarding, 111–12
soccer team, women's national, 42
social facilitation, 22
social media attention, 12, 124–25
So Many Olympic Exertions (Chen), 189–90
South Asians in Sports networking group, 43
Speak Your Mind podcast, 146
Sport, Rhetoric, and Political Struggle (Schuck), 65–66
Sport and the Sociological Imagination (Lerch), 189
Sport and the Sociological Imagination (Rosenberg), 188
Sports Illustrated, 5, 17, 39, 45, 46, 47, 71, 74, 76, 89, 102, 105, 114, 115, 125, 139, 147, 150, 152, 153, 154, 155, 156, 178, 186, 187, 197, 200, 205
Stamatis, Andreas, 5
Stanford soccer, 130
Steinbrecher, Jon, 128–29

Steinfort, Paddy, 39–40, 47–48, 51, 54–56
Sterrett, John E., 28, 30
Stewart, Breanna, 182
Stills, Kenny, 152–53, 155
St. Louis Browns, 31–34
Street, Picabo, 180–81
Stroop test, 47
Studies from the Yale Psychological Laboratory, 23
substance use: alcohol, 140, 146–49; athletes' similarities to people with addictions, 142; cannabis consumption, 143–45; Carcillo's experience with, 139–41; culture of, 141–43; drug testing, 143–45, 155; Lehner on, 84; most common, 143; rehabilitation centers for, 147–49; self-medication, 142–43
Sudano, Laura, 123
suicide: athletes placed on watch for, 88; attempts at, 62, 74–76, 133; college athletes' rates of, 7; football players and, 3–4, 156; in NCAA, 129–32; Olympic athletes and, 17–18. *See also* depression
"sweet spot" in performing, 51–52
Świątek, Iga, 46
swimmers. *See* Phelps, Michael
Symonds, Anna, 151, 152, 155

Taking MACtion Summit, 128

Taylor, Garrett, 139

Teammates for Mental Health, 128

Ted Lasso (TV show), 18

telehealth providers, 121

tennis, 7, 109–11. *See also specific athletes*

The Sideline Perspective blog, 13

Thomas, Louisa, xx

Thomas, Solomon, 187

"thoughts aren't facts," 52

Till the End (Sabathia and Smith), 147

time-off from games: benefits, 191–92; challenges of rehabilitation, 182–83; during COVID-19, 185–87; grieving process, 177–78, 181; identity loss with, 177–79; need for, 93–94; retirement and professional help, 184–85; retirement as "social death," 188–89; stepping back before retirement, 187–88

Tissié, Philippe, 22–23

Tokyo Olympics, xix–xx, 89, 105, 107, 111–12, 186–87

Toronto Blue Jays, 52

Toronto Raptors, 79

Tracy, David F., 30–34

Treadway, Caroline, 163, 165

Treating Athletes with Eating Disorders (Bennett), 161–62

triage, 50–51

Triplett, Norman, 22

Trujillo, Natasha, 164, 170, 174, 176

trust, 51–52

Tulsa Shock, 88

twisties, 105–6

Twitter, 79–80

Uberoi, Neha, 43, 45

UFC (Ultimate Fighting Championship), 151, 154

Ultimate Fighting Championship (UFC), 151, 154

UNCUT, 132–33

unionization of student athletes, 37–38, 134

UNIT3D podcast, 16

University of Colorado Boulder, 178

University of Connecticut, 125

University of Minnesota, 181

University of North Texas, 125

USA Gymnastics statements, 104–5

U.S. Olympic and Paralympic Committee (USOPC), 38, 112–14, 178, 184–85

Utah Jazz, 185

Vanderbilt soccer, 125

Van Slingerland, Krista, xxii

VanVleet, Fred, 80

Vealey, Robin, 35

Vecsey, George, 148

Veeck, William, 29, 30

Victory Program, 174, 175

visualization exercises,
48–49. *See also* mindfulness and
meditation
vulnerability, 9–10

WADA (World Anti-Doping
Agency), 143–44, 155
Wall, John, 86
Walton, Courtney Campbell,
150–51
Wambach, Abby, 13
Washington Mystics, 62
Washington State football, 117,
121. *See also* Hilinski, Tyler
(and family)
Washington Wizards, 83
The Weight of Gold (documentary),
17, 75–76, 113
Welch, Bob, 148–49
Wertheim, L. Jon, 71, 115
Wesana Health, 153–54
Whalen, Eamon, 73
What Made Maddy Run (Fagan),
10, 125, 130
Wheeler, Benjamin Ide, 6

Where Tomorrows Aren't Promised
(Anthony), 9–10
White, Royce, 70–73, 141–42
Wiener, William, 182–83
Williams, Caleb, 126
Williams, Serena, 99, 100, 114–15,
182–83
Williams, Venus, 114–15
WNBA (Women's National
Basketball Association), 93, 102
Women and Sport (Oglesby), 36
Women's National Basketball
Association (WNBA), 93, 102
World Anti-Doping Agency
(WADA), 143–44, 155
Wrigley, Philip K., 28–30
Wrigleyville (Golenbock), 28–29

Yang, Melissa, 94
Yates, Dorothy Hazeltine, 35, 36
Yazar-Klosinski, Berra, 153
Yurchenko, Natalia, 104

Zeta-Jones, Catherine, 61–62
Zuppke, Robert, 26–27

About the Author

Julie Kliegman has been copy chief at *Sports Illustrated*, copy editor at *The Ringer*, weekend editor at *The Week*, and news fellow at *BuzzFeed*. Her writing as appeared in *Sports Illustrated*, the *Washington Post*, *The Ringer*, *Vulture*, *BuzzFeed*, *Vox*, *The Verge*, *Bustle*, *Washington Monthly*, *The Week*, and more. Kliegman is a frequent guest on radio and podcasts. She lives in Queens, New York, with her cat, Penelope.